AS KINKY AS YOU WANNA BE

YOUR GUIDE TO SAFE, SANE AND SMART BDSM

SHANNA GERMAIN

CLEiS
PRESS

Published in the United States by Cleis Press, Inc., 2246 Sixth Street, Berkeley, California 94710.

Printed in the United States.
Cover design: Scott Idleman/Blink
Cover photograph: iStockphoto
Text design: Frank Wiedemann

First Edition.
10 9 8 7 6 5 4 3 2 1

Trade paper ISBN: 978-1-62778-062-9
E-book ISBN: 978-1-62778-074-2

CONTENTS

CONTENTS

INTRODUCTION:
THE WONDERFUL WORLD OF KINK

D earest Reader,

Welcome to the wonderful world of kink!

Chances are, if you're reading this book, this isn't your first foray into kink country. Maybe you've had a few experiences here and there. Maybe you've seen a movie or read a novel full of hair pulling, spanking and "yes, pleases." Or maybe you're an expert in getting it on, kinky style.

Whether it's your first time or thousandth adventure: welcome. Come on in, buckle up and have a seat. We're about to take a wild ride.

Before we get started, here's what you should know about this book: *As Kinky as You Wanna Be* isn't a hands-on, how-to book. It won't teach you how to build a crop, tie ropes around your squirming lover or choose the proper lube. Don't get me wrong—books like that are an important part of any sexual education, especially a kinky one, and there are many, many wonderful books like that already available. In fact, in the back of this book you'll find a Resource Guide (page 176) with some of my favorites. I recommend that you stock at least a few of them in your sex library (and if you don't have a sex library already, I recommend one of those too—there's nothing more wonderful than having a collection of great books on hand for just the right learning opportunity).

This book, however, is designed to do something different. Rather than provide a hands-on how-to where you're getting up close and personal with an intimate aspect of BDSM, such as tying knots or sampling nipple clamps, this book invites you to step back and take a broader view. Consider it a travel guide to BDSM, if you will. Or perhaps a road map to your own kinky self. Follow this path to adventures unexplored, to the beautiful scrape of a nail across skin, to the smell of leather and lust, to the low moans of someone in the very midst of pleasure.

In this book, you're invited to explore the wonderful world of kink—and perhaps more importantly, to discover your own personal pleasure spots along the way. What does your kinky landscape look like? What is the language of this world that you're about to enter? How do you navigate the customs and rituals of the BDSM community? *As Kinky as You Wanna Be* guides you through all of these terrains, and more.

Along the way, you'll also have the opportunity to hear experts talk about everything from exploring self-identity to staying healthy to playing well with others. Shanna Katz gives us her expert tips for communicating about kink, while Sunny Megatron goes wild about the joys of toys. Need to prepare for emergencies? Jay Wiseman has just what the doctor ordered, while Dr. Lynk tells you how to keep your body healthy and well for whatever dirty activities you can dream up.

But this book offers more than expert advice—it also offers a whole slew of delicious kinky stories from some of the industry's best fiction writers, designed to whet your appetite and spark your kinky creativity. Let these talented writers show you the way to your own debauchery. Want to scream "Oh god!" in your favorite church along with the main character in Remittance Girl's story, "Amanda, Agnus Dei"? Or perhaps a little public dominance and submission, á la Rachel Kramer Bussel's "Petting Zoo," is more your style. Go along for the virtual ride with Stella Harris's sexy take on "The Only Real Girl on the Internet," or get out of breath watching the lovers play power games in "Bearers," by Nikki Magennis. Even during the roughest times, kinky sex can be the light that saves us; my own story, "The Sun Is an Ordinary Star," shows us a couple using kink to get through a life-changing event, while Kristina Lloyd breaks all the taboos in her story, "The Wrong Woman," to remind us just how hot a dirty, naughty fantasy can be. Lastly, this book includes places to Get Your Passport Stamped—experiences to try and new avenues to explore to broaden your kinky horizons. Don't be afraid to try them out and see how they feel. You might be surprised to discover how perfectly some of these new experiences fit, almost as if they were custom-made for your very pleasure.

Bondage, submission, dominance, pain and pleasure—you'll find it all within these pages. All you have to do is take that first step.

So what are we waiting for? Let's kick off this luscious, lovely kinky adventure!

Yours in kinkaliciousness,
Shanna Germain

CHAPTER ONE

DISCOVERING YOUR KINKY LANDSCAPE

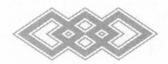

Not that many years ago, I was sitting in a coffee shop with an erotica-writer friend of mine. I was leaving for a year-long trip around the world, so this was the last time we were going to see each other for a while. We were talking about all aspects of our lives, and the conversation eventually turned to sex. (You'd think we would get there quicker, being erotica writers and all, but sometimes after writing about sex all day, the last thing you want to talk about is sex. I suppose it's one of the hazards of the job.)

I can't remember what she said that prompted me to say the following, but I will never forget saying it: "I'm a total pain slut."

Yes, I said that, right in the middle of the coffee shop.

I thought she might choke on her coffee and fall over right there. But the truth was, I was as surprised as she was that I'd said it.

Not because we were in public or because I was uncomfortable telling her, but because until the very moment the words came out of my mouth, I hadn't known that it was true. I had known that my sexuality was changing, that I was evolving—I could feel it happening—but it took an open-minded friend creating a safe place before I could speak the truth that was brewing in the back of my mind, before I could discover this new identity.

Even from a young age, I knew that I was attracted to people of all genders, that sometimes I liked being told what to do or what to say, and that being around intelligent people was a huge turn-on. My mind didn't have access to words like *omnisexual, submissive,* or *sapiosexual* until much later, but my heart and body had already told me, in no uncertain terms, some of the things it liked.

My tastes—and certainly my vocabulary—have grown a lot since then, but one thing that's stayed constant is that I still have a wide variety of sexual interests and identities.

BDSM. Kinky. Vanilla. Dominant. Submissive. Top. Bottom. Pain slut...

These are words that get thrown around a lot, especially today, thanks to the increasing popularity of novels and films that explore these themes in myriad ways. But what do those words mean? And more importantly: what do they mean to you?

All you have to do is search any of the above terms on the Internet, and you'll quickly discover that they mean something almost completely different to each person who uses them. It's easy to get overwhelmed with options: Spanking. Being spanked. Bondage. Hair pulling. Forced chastity. Exhibitionism. Anal sex. Role-play. The list goes on and on. (It really does—for even more options, check out the Fetishes and Interests section of the Glossary, starting on page 167. And that's just a sample of the most popular options.)

What if you just like a little hair pulling or a dirty whisper from time to time? Or you get hot at the idea of being spanked by a sexy woman, but you've never actually tried it? Or maybe you're just not sure about all of it, but you'd like to learn more.

Does that mean you're kinky?

Sure, why not? In my opinion, kink is a label that encompasses much more than it leaves out, from a tantalizing striptease with your spouse to a full-on play party full of bondage and butt plugs; kinky pretty much covers it all.

According to the general definition, kinky means any activity that is "marked by unconventional sexual preferences or behavior." The tricky part about that is actually defining "unconventional." Is premarital sex unconventional? It is in some parts of the world. Does that mean it's kinky? Maybe. What about anal sex, a threesome, dirty talk or playing doctor? What if your interests—say you like to be tossed over someone's knee and spanked until you cry—don't actually involve any sexual activities? Is that kinky? Again, the answer probably varies widely, depending on cultural norms and your own boundaries and expectations.

Perhaps a better way to define kink doesn't focus so much on the activities as it does the attitudes. In its most basic, broadest sense, we could define kink as a gift box, containing multitudes of desires and needs, all wrapped up with a pretty bow of power exchange. You can give the gift to yourself, or you can share it with the one(s) you love or lust for. That part is up to you.

At a deeper level, I think of kink as being a term that we can use to talk about any type of intimate, consensual exchange of power between people. If we think of it that way, kink encompasses a huge variety of people, practices, experiences and cultures—anyone and anything that stretches the boundaries of sex beyond the traditional norms and explores the unexplored.

So, what's the appeal? Why do people get kinky?

Because it turns them on, of course!

But that's only a small part of it.

People who practice kink do it for any number of reasons: to test and stretch their limits, to conquer fears or anxieties, to experience something wholly new, to walk the fine line between pain and pleasure or for some purpose that is wholly their own.

Sometimes those experiences are physical. Other times they are spiritual, mental, erotic, sensual or a combination of all of these. Being kinky isn't always about sex. Someone who gets off on pain, for example, may feel a sexual release when he is spanked by someone else, or a submissive may find it relaxing and arousing when she is dominated by her partner, but they may not think of it as being about sex at all.

Here's the important thing about words and their definitions: no one else is more of an expert on yourself than you are. If you say you are [fill in the blank], then you are.

But how do you know what you are? And what if it keeps changing?

Uncertainty and change are both normal, healthy parts of being a human being, whether we're talking about our career choices, our living arrangements or our sexual identities. But sometimes, especially when we're in the midst of trying to figure things out and get answers, it's easy to forget that. The same is true with our sexual identities. Not only do our sexual interests and desires change over time, so does the way that we perceive sex and ourselves as sexual creatures. And, believe it or not, that's a good thing.

As award-winning author and sex educator Tristan Taormino writes in her book *The Ultimate Guide to Kink: BDSM, Role Play and the Erotic Edge*, "Exploring kink provides us with an opportunity for self-reflection, challenge, and personal growth. Where many people are content to just sit back and let life happen, we're not: we constantly engage our identities, sexualities, and relationships."

I'm no longer the person I once was, the girl who surprised her friend—and herself—by publicly declaring she was a pain slut. My sexual interests have changed yet again. On any given day, my turn-ons are a little bit from Column A, a little bit from Column B and a lot from Column Whatever I Feel Like That Day. And that, for me, is the perfect route to a kinky sex life.

Get Your Passport Stamped: Find Your Turn-Ons

Some of us know right away where our kinky interests lie. If the thought of having your ass smacked with a leather paddle leaves you gasping and wet, you can pretty much take a guess on at least one kinky thing that might interest you.

Others of us aren't sure. Thankfully, self-discovery can be an exciting and arousing aspect of being a kinky person. Here are some directions you might want to explore.

1. Make Sense of Your Senses

One of the things that you'll first learn about yourself is what senses are most stimulating for you. How you like your kink to be served up can be almost as important as what your kink actually is.

Even as a writer and reader of erotica, I find that most of my erotic inspiration comes from visual images. I like to see (and, in the case of videos, hear) what's happening—how light plays off damp skin, what rope looks like when it's slowly wound around a pair of wrists, how someone sounds when he or she is begging for more. A large part of power play for me is, perhaps not surprisingly given my profession, the words that come with it.

When I teach erotica writing classes, I often tell my students to imagine that their characters are most strongly driven by one of the five senses. If a character is visual, her sexuality will be focused on what she can see. She'll describe things visually, and even use words like "I see your point" to describe non-visual elements. On the other hand, someone who's auditory will be focused on sounds—the light slap of palm to skin, the words that someone speaks, the way breath rises and falls. He will say things like "I hear what you're saying" to show that he's listening.

This is probably true of all of us. Most of us have one or more dominant senses (and contrary to popular belief, your sense of choice probably has very little to do with your gender). While knowing your dominant sense(s) doesn't define your kink, it can have a huge impact on how much you enjoy it. Submissives with a strong auditory bent will want to hear their partner say those sensual words of power, while those with a stronger visual sensibility might enjoy watching themselves be dominated in front of a mirror.

2. What's Your Hot Button?

There are so many options when it comes to kinky activities that it would be nearly impossible to make a comprehensive list. Despite the wide array, it's pretty likely that you already know at least one or two things that really speak to you. Many people discover their kinks early on and often by accident—wrestling with a friend suddenly opens up a lifelong love of naked grappling with partners, the soft touch of a partner's stockings sends you over the edge, an accidental tangle in the bedsheets while masturbating turns into a full-on bondage fetish. Other lucky ones discover their kinks through the help of their partners—a quick slap on the butt during sex or a bit of dominance play in a safe environment is sometimes all it takes to open the fetish floodgates.

But what if you want to know more? Or what if you have an idea that there's something out there for you, but you don't know what it is? One of the easiest ways to explore your own kinky side is to read a wide selection of erotic literature or look at myriad sexy videos or images. With public libraries stocking erotica collections and a proliferation of fetish sites on the web, it has never been easier and more inexpensive to discover your own kinks in a private, low-stress way. As you read or look, pay special attention to the elements that make your breath catch and get your heart pounding. Watch and read as widely as you can. (Yes, I'm giving you permission to go a little sex crazy! If someone gives you a hard time about it, you can point right to this paragraph and say, "Look, right here. She said to read and watch as much as I could.")

Keep a turn-on journal. Write stories or snippets of fantasies. Use a place like Pinterest or Tumblr to gather sexy images. Not only will these activities help you solidify your own kinks, they could be a useful tool in the future, when it's time to start talking about kinks to your partner(s) (see Chapter Two: Talking the Talk for more information on this).

3. What's Your Off Button?

As you're exploring, don't just note what turns you on. Also think about the things that don't do anything for you and the activities that you actively don't like. While your turnoffs (sometimes called *soft limits*—things that you don't find arousing, but that you might be willing to try with the right partner or in the right situation) and your definite nos (sometimes called *hard limits*—things that you aren't willing to do or interested in doing under any circumstances, or things that are clearly dangerous to you) might change over time, it's good to have a starting place for your interests. Keep a list of turnoffs, but don't be surprised if they are less rigid than you expect. Sometimes when you start exploring kink, you discover that there's a whole lot more to like than you originally thought.

4. Take the Plunge—Carefully

Did you find your fetish? Can't wait to go out and buy a set of leather handcuffs or try your hand at a little wax play? Great. It's time for the next step: turning your fantasy into reality.

When it comes to BDSM, it's always best to share your experiences with someone you know well, trust completely and can communicate with in an honest way. This is especially true of your first time. Nothing can sour your own self-exploration faster than a negative or scary experience.

If you already have a willing partner that you trust, it's time to start talking about expectations and desires and go from there.

If, on the other hand, you're still looking for that perfect someone (or someones) who share your interests, it's a good idea to go slow. Even if you're pretty sure you're going to pass out from excitement if you don't get to try out your new fascination with blindfolds RIGHT NOW, take a deep breath and a step back. Read the chapters in this book on health and safety. You want to make sure your first experience is safe, positive, supportive—and, of course, hot as well. How else will you know just how much you like it?

YOU CONTAIN MULTITUDES:

Cecilia Tan on Self-Identity

Cecilia Tan claims the titles of writer, editor and activist, and that's just for starters. "You could throw event organizer, educator, public speaker, fundraiser and a bunch of other things into that list, too," she says. "When you're an activist, you see a need, you fill it. I didn't expect to become the founder/organizer of the largest BDSM/leather/fetish event in New England, but I did, because no one else would take me up on my suggestion that we should have a Fetish Flea Market."

You've known you were kinky since you were very young. How did you find your own way into your kinky self?

I would say my kink exploration started when I was five or six years old and was focused on a lot of "let's pretend" around the old *Batman* TV series. Catwoman was so obviously a kinky template, even for a five-year-old who didn't know what it was about. She ties Batman up and seduces him—even in the kids' TV show! In the comic books she has high heels and a whip and everything. I always assumed, though, as I grew up, that if I wanted to bring that kind of "let's pretend" into the actual bedroom, I was going to have to start from scratch convincing each partner of mine to give it a try. Then when I graduated college I moved to Boston and discovered the leather community and the alt. sex.bondage newsgroup on the fledgling Internet (1990). Boom, I was suddenly in touch with thousands and thousands of people all over the world who were kinky and practiced BDSM. And when I say practiced I mean really practiced to get it right! These folks took classes on how to flog and tie people up. These folks TAUGHT classes on how to flog and tie people up. I jumped into the community with both feet as an activist—writing, teaching, organizing, fundraising, founding groups and events, et cetera, and here we are twenty-something years later.

For those just beginning to explore their own kinky side, what advice can you give about the process?

I think people tend to look for labels that fit. Rope top, sissy maid, Daddy, masochist, et cetera. I think labels can be useful as a kind of shorthand when you're trying to meet people and connect—think about how personal ads work—but it's important to realize that for most people there's no one single label that encapsulates their identity. At first it's so freeing to declare "I'm a (slave/Master/puppy)!" because normal society doesn't want you to. But it can be restricting and stultifying to feel now that you've declared it, that's ALL you can be. And while there is a lot to learn from mentors, don't let anyone tell you there's only one "right" way to be a Master, slave, puppy, or whatever. It's between you and your play partners or your relationships to define for yourselves what the "right" way is. I'm a classic example. I just celebrated my twenty-second anniversary with Corwin. We were both known as heavy masochists in our BDSM social circle when we went on a date with each other, and people were like "Whut? But you're both bottoms? What are you gonna DO?" Fact is, we're both switches, but people forget that people can switch the way they forget that bisexuals exist. So my advice is remember you contain multitudes and don't let anyone's "rules" stop you from exploring yourself or other people.

As a writer yourself, do you think that writing is a good way for people to gain a better understanding of their own desires and interests?

Absolutely. I used to teach a class at adult education centers about freeing the erotic imagination through writing. (I'd still be teaching it, but I'm too busy writing!) These days whether you just write dirty tweets and sexts to the one person you want to turn on, or whether you start a "secret life of anonymous" blog, or you decide to do National Novel Writing Month, there's no "wrong" way to explore fantasies. I also think reading erotica is an underrated form of exploration. Reading is the ultimate safe sex. You can try out all kinds of fetishes and experiences and get an idea of whether they map to your inner desires or not, all from the comfort of your armchair (or bed).

Some people's sexual and gender identity never changes, but for others, it's an ever-evolving process—we grow older, our experiences or partners change us, our bodies change, and so on.

Can you talk a little about your own experience with this and what you learned from it?

Since I started out a bisexual switch to begin with, maybe I'm more mutable than others, or maybe I just have much wider tastes. I've definitely evolved both in what turns me on and in what my sexual "identity" is. I used to really be a smart-assed masochist; I was into heavy-duty pain and being challenged by it and in challenging the authority of the top who had to put me in my place. After I had a back injury, though, my conception of myself as indestructible changed, and that desire to test my pain threshold waned. I also went through a bad breakup at one point with a top who had brought out my "loyal submissive" side, so breaking up with him made it pretty impossible to pursue those kinds of relationships. In life, things happen outside your control. Sometimes they're things you do by choice, like people who become vegetarians for reasons of conscience or those who decide to eat more nuts for their health; other times you have no choice, like people who develop gluten sensitivity. It's funny: many people seem to accept easily that as we grow and change, what we eat will change, but they don't accept that our erotic appetites and needs may change just as drastically. In the erotica writing world we have the phrase "bulletproof kink" to describe the one thing that will get a particular person hot regardless of the quality of the story (or lack thereof) or what kind of mood they're in. Truth is, most readers have few bulletproof kinks that work every time for their whole lives.

Sometimes, when we "come out" as one thing and then grow and realize we've become something else, we experience strong emotions from our loved ones.

What are some methods for handling this transition in a positive way for both our own needs and the needs of those we are close to?

Message to everyone's loved ones: the map is not the territory. The label is not the person. A bisexual friend married her girlfriend recently and her mother wanted to know if that meant now she had "become" a lesbian. She had to explain, no Mom, I'm actually still a bisexual, I'm just monogamous now. I know it can be confusing to people who live in a privileged, sheltered box where they think everyone they know is heterosexual and vanilla like themselves and the perceived majority. The nonstandard labels become something they can cling to without having to actually work to understand what those labels mean. It's frustrating, but each person has to decide what level of engagement with their loved ones (and the mainstream in general) to have about his or her sexual identity.

On the one hand, yes, we need more people to be out and open about erotic needs and sexual truths. Coming out is incredibly important for that reason. The only reason systematic sexual abuse can take place is because people don't talk about sex and are taught not to talk about sex, even the good sex.

On the other hand, for most people, their sex life really isn't anyone's business. Is it anyone's job as a minority (of any kind) to educate the majority about him or her self? It gets tiring and can be soul-killing to always be the one having to explain everything about being the only Asian in a group, or the only lesbian, or the only trans person, or the only blind person. (Or the only writer…) In my case, I've pretty much made it my life's work to try to explain and validate the existence of erotic minorities, but that's at least partly so other people won't have to! Yes, it's a drag when you spend a decade trying to get your mom to accept that you're bisexual and to understand what that means, only to have her ask if you're a lesbian now that you're married. It's probably even more of a drag for people who actually DO feel they've shifted from one thing to another, from one label class to another. Even the most supportive families can be invested in your former label: "What do you mean you're not a lesbian anymore? Does this mean I can't wear my PROUD MOTHER OF A LESBIAN shirt to Pride Day anymore?" I try to distance the conversation from the personal to the linguistic structures that force us to place these labels where we do, and to get people to understand that the labels are arbitrary. Maybe there's some other label that would have encompassed both what I was and what I now am, and in some other system of division, some other society or some other planet, perhaps, that would make perfect sense and not be confusing. Then again, I've got a degree in linguistics, so of course I look at it that way. Labels, like words, are only an approximation of their underlying meaning, a consensual cluster of ideology such that if you start asking people "What does this word mean?", the discussion quickly diverges into "everyone has a different definition" anyway. Words, and sexualities, are slippery like that.

What question has no one ever asked you on this topic, but you wish someone would?

Ooh, tricky! How about "What is your bulletproof kink and why is it the thing that always works for you?"

What's your answer to that question?

Even more tricky! Damn, now I have to come up with the answer. Okay, given that I have such wide-ranging tastes in people, partners and pornography, I have to say I think my bulletproof kink is willing self-sacrifices. Sexual self-sacrifices, I should clarify. You know, the "we have to have sex to save the world" sorts of scenarios. I have no idea why this is my thing, though. Maybe that's the definition of a bulletproof kink, though: I don't know why I like it, it JUST WORKS.

AMANDA, AGNUS DEI

Remittance Girl

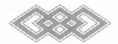

I walked Amanda up the worn stone steps of St. James's Church in Spanish Place, beneath the shadows of its uncanny gargoyles and into the cool, dark interior. Her arm muscles twitched in my grip. The tendons of her neck stood out like wires. I loved her like this.

"You can do this, sweet."

She bobbed her head but said nothing. She didn't have to. I knew she was scared. Knew that the familiar reek of stale incense and floor polish, the stench of hypocrisy and Holy Ghost were worming their way into her pores, corroding her courage.

What a paradox it is, to despise how Amanda allowed this crap to eat away at her self-worth and yet still be unbelievably turned on by how vulnerable it rendered her. Call it arrogance, hubris or just a greed for control, but I didn't want to compete with the whole of the mother Church. If she had to be vulnerable, I wanted to be the one who made her feel that way. Not a fucking institution.

When I caught her, like I have caught her often, on her knees with her hands clasped together, fingers interlaced and white with desperation, weeping into the duvet, I thought, *Fuck this. This has got to stop.*

She wasn't crying for me. She was wracked by guilt for what we do: the things she loves me to do to her, the despicable perversions that turn her tendons to jelly and make her come so hard. She wept over the exquisite creature she becomes when I render her fuck meat. When I punish her ass with my hand. When she raises her hips like a frantic cat in heat and soaks my fingers.

So, if I was forced to compete with that prick up there above the altar, I decided there was no remedy but to take it to the source.

"Over there," I said, urging her to a pew halfway down the nave, facing the chancel.

The old wood creaked as we sat, side by side, in the deserted, sepulchral cave. St. James was the darkest church I could find. It was usually empty during the week and there were rumors that it would soon close due to its aging and dwindling congregation. I entertained the fantasy of buying it and turning it into the kink club of my dreams. Not very likely, but it was a kick-ass daydream.

There he was, pendant in all his über-masochistic glory. My dominance usurped by the biggest sub of all times. That's the other reason I had chosen St. James. The central crucifixion was luxuriantly obscene. His crown of thorns was vicious; rivulets of lurid red striped his pallid wooden face. The nails in his palms could never have held his bodyweight in reality; they'd have ripped right through his hands. But there they were, pinning him to a stylized tree. The wounds in his side seeped a darker fluid, and his heart was exposed and glowing. His groin cloth-wrapped, sexless.

"Kneel." I shoved over one of the burgundy leather pads that dotted the kneeler with the toe of my shoe.

Amanda hesitated.

I turned, slipped my arm around her shoulders and nestled my mouth against her ear. "Kneel, or I'll drag you up to the altar by your hair, bend you over it and fuck your ass. No lube."

She tried to pull away from me. "Someone could come in. Someone could see," she hissed.

"Look at me, Amanda. Do you think I care? Do you think I'm not perfectly willing to take whatever the consequences of that might be? At worst I'd be charged with lewd and indecent behavior. Chances are, they'd just freak out and tell us to leave." I stared at her face. "I'm not the one worried about my immortal soul, my sweet. And I don't believe God gives a shit where I fuck your ass."

"Sh-sh!" She took panicked, furtive glances around the church. Then it sank in. She read my face and knew I was telling her the absolute truth. My threat wasn't idle. "Okay. Okay!"

Amanda edged off the pew, onto her knees. She wore a mid-length blue cotton dress dappled with tiny white fleur-de-lis. It snugged in at her waist, flared at her magnificent hips and draped over her generous ass, catching in the crease of her buttocks. She'd followed my instructions to leave the panties at home.

If there was ever a woman worthy to pose for a likeness of the Virgin Mary, it was Amanda. So scrumptiously female. Not just feminine but female. Fleshy in all the right places. Haunches that begged grabbing, breasts that demanded mauling. Asscheeks that took a slap and reverberated pleasingly with the force of it. The plumpest, juiciest cunt I'd ever buried my cock in. I'm not saying I could never love an anorexic woman, but it was a lot easier to love Amanda.

Behind her on the pew, I reached forward and trailed my knuckles down her spine. "Put your hands together and pray."

"What...what should I pray for?"

The curve of her ass was warm through the fabric. She twitched and straightened her back, pressed her palms together and interlaced her fingers.

"I don't care. It's not going to matter in about five minutes."

Beneath the skirt, the backs of her bare thighs were buttery soft. I made a wedge of my hand and pushed my way between them, into the heat and the pressure. She clenched her legs together with such ferocity it took considerable effort to reach her cunt.

Instead of asking, because she knew exactly what I wanted, I caught a nice soft piece of inner thigh between two fingers and pinched her hard enough to elicit a gasp.

"I can't," she whispered.

"You can. You will."

I pinched again, in exactly the same spot, hard enough to leave an ugly bruise. But I like ugly bruises. It gives me a reason to kiss them better. She didn't release the tension in her thighs, but she edged her knees apart, just enough to afford me access to what I wanted.

Soft and smooth and humid, the entrance to Amanda's grave cave was the source of most of her misery and a good deal of her joy. She was too scared to be truly wet, but Amanda had a well that never really ran dry. I eased my fingertips between her ripe lips and into her smooth, humid slit.

I buried my face in the abundance of her dark hair and whispered. "I hope you're praying."

"N-noooo." More of a bleat than a word.

Little Lamb of God Amanda. Who turns me inside out with her brimming eyes and her flooding cunt. Who validates every nasty thing I do to her by orgasming louder than anyone I've ever been with.

I shifted the angle of my hand, pressing the edges of it into the taut and trembling tendons that attempted, with or without intention, to keep me out. She fought and she fought and then, pressing her forehead to her clasped hands, she relented and relaxed her thighs.

"Thank you, sweet."

Her internal muscles fluttered as I probed her hole with my middle finger. The interior of her cunt was like a cat's tongue, and I've never been able to fuck her with my fingers without having my cock swell at the texture. She was smooth and rough, tight and accommodating all at the same time.

Now she was all tensed up and only just moist enough for me to penetrate. But I knew Amanda. It wouldn't be this way for long.

"You know what you want, Amanda."

The knuckles of her joined fingers were white. Lips bitten together, the way they started out when I laid a first hard blow on her ass.

"Mmmm."

It wasn't a moan of pleasure, but the muted sound of a whimper. I held my hand still, my finger embedded and motionless. I read her interior war in the jagged contractions around it.

"Be brave, my gorgeous girl. Come on. You know what you want."

For a very long moment—an eon in which I had time to wonder if I'd made a very bad mistake—she knelt there like a statue, as seized up on the inside as she looked on the outside.

Maybe I didn't understand her after all? Maybe I'd convinced myself this would be good for her because it was what I wanted. Maybe I had no fucking business coming between her and her God. Maybe I was just an arrogant prick?

I thought about removing my hand. I thought about the humiliation of patting her on the shoulder and saying: "Okay, sorry, love. I've made a mistake." I wrestled with the consequences of that: of being wrong in her eyes, of heedlessly pushing her where she just couldn't go.

Then, she inhaled—drank in the musty, incense-bitter air in a long, low, stuttered breath—and began to move her hips.

It wasn't until that moment I noticed how dry my throat had

grown. The rush of relief burned my chest and sent a spike of lust through my groin. Instantly, I was hard and throbbing.

"There's my good girl," I whispered, brushing her long hair to one side and tracing her cheek with my free hand.

"Oh, god!" She choked on the words and pushed her ass backward, forcing more of my finger into her heat.

She did it again, and again: tiny little backward movements at first, but then her cunt began to weep around my finger, until she slid herself easily onto it and my palm was slick with her juices.

I watched her hips grind, listened to her breath roughen, but her eyes were shut tight and that wouldn't do. She imagined herself somewhere else, I was sure of it.

"Open your eyes, Amanda. Open them."

"No," she protested. But there was no heart behind it and a familiar twist curved her lips. The crooked smile she always wore in pleasure.

I angled my hand and forced in a second digit. "Do it! Look at him."

She snatched a breath and her lids flashed open. Wide, staring, scared and aroused. But it didn't stop her from moving. She was still, relentlessly, fucking herself on my fingers.

I slipped my free hand under her jaw and pulled her head up. "Look at him, Amanda. He's too damn busy dying to love you like I do."

She hiccuped a sob. I felt it against my fingers, like something ripped from her throat. Below, the first tentative contractions announced an impending orgasm. Her hips moved fluidly, with a mindless intentionality.

"He's never going to love your suffering the way I love it. Never."

Tears began to course down her cheeks. Her entire body trembled. Slicking my thumb in the sopping mess between her legs, I pressed it into her ass.

"No...no..." she gasped.

I wasn't sure whether she was agreeing with me or was whining about my penetration of her tighter, darker hole. And I didn't care.

I hauled her back from the rail and plunged my fingers into her with all my strength. "He can't make you come like I can."

She stiffened in my arm, jerked once, twice, and came with such force I thought she'd squeeze my fingers out of their sockets. It went on and on: eyes wide and fixed on that hanging abomination while her fluids covered over my hand and trickled down the insides of her legs.

"Fuck..." she croaked. "Fuck you!"

I didn't have to ask. I knew who she was talking to. Her gaze was pinned to the Christ above the altar. And there was a blazing anger in those eyes. Even as the last of her contractions tugged my fingers, as she gave a hard shudder in my arm, she said it again.

"Fuck you. Fuck you. Fuck you."

I freed my hand and smoothed the back of her dress down, then pulled her off her knees and onto my lap.

We sat in silence for a while, listening to the pews around us creak as they expanded in the afternoon heat. I smiled at her musky scent. It completely overpowered the acrid smell of the incense. She cuddled against my chest for a long while and then pulled back to look up at me.

"I'm so insanely hungry." Her hand snaked into my lap and she rubbed her open palm against the bulge in my pants. "I could suck your cock in an alley, then we could find somewhere to eat."

I growled. "No, I'm hungry too. Eat first, fuck later," I said, getting to my feet and pulling her up with me.

As we walked out of St. James's and into the early afternoon light, we almost collided with a wizened old priest on rickety legs, climbing the front steps.

"Good afternoon!"

I smiled and nodded. "Afternoon, Father."

"So nice to see young people coming back to the Church," he said. His ancient, mottled hand gripped the wrought-iron railing and he continued his ascent.

CHAPTER TWO

TALKING THE TALK

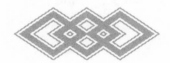

W hat's the hardest part about kinky sex? Ask this question at any BDSM-themed event or gathering and you'll get a lot of answers, often accompanied by a fair amount of laughter and giggling.

"Trying to find a safe place to hide the sex toys from the kids."

"Answering the important phone call from my boss while trussed up like a turkey."

"Figuring out just the *right* way to pinch my submissive's nipples to make him scream."

While those are all certainly difficult—some, in fact, require great skill, great patience and no shortage of luck to pull off—perhaps the hardest kinky act is simply this: talking about it openly and honestly.

Sadly, we don't live in a culture that encourages open, frank conversations about even the very basics of sex, much less the complicated topics that kink can bring to the bedroom (or playroom). So those of us who are kinky need to go that extra step when talking about our desires and interests. And that makes it even more difficult. Not talking about our sexual interests is a dangerous loop that is hard—but not impossible—to break.

Why can it be so hard to broach the subject of kink with our partners or prospective partners? We all know the answer to that. Fear of rejection. Fear of being laughed at. Fear of being considered "weird" or "gross." Fear of losing or turning off the ones we love.

Fear. Fear. Fear. Often accompanied by shame, guilt, anxiety, insecurity and a million other awful, gut-wrenching feelings that try to convince us to keep our mouths shut, hide our passions and pretend yet again that we're perfectly happy with things the way they are—even when we know that the way things are is a slow, quiet killer of sexual passion.

Finding a way to move past these negative feelings is the first step in truly talking about your wants and needs, and boy is that first step a doozy. So let me hold out my hand and help you get over it right now by saying this: Someone's going to laugh at you. Someone's going to think you're weird. Someone's going to run away screaming when you tell him that your greatest fantasy is to be humiliated in public or cuffed to the bed and screwed senseless.

That someone is not for you.

I know: it's easy for me to say that from here, when I'm not the one with important things at stake. Families. Marriages. Relationships. Stability. Security. Love. Whether or not to take that risk is something that only you can decide.

But I've been there. I've had partners who I loved deeply and shared my life with, and I had to choose whether or not to have this conversation with them, knowing that I was potentially risking everything we'd built together. The vast majority of those conversations went better than I expected, often opening the door for my partners to start talking about *their* unmet sexual needs. This happens more often than you might think; even as you're worrying about expressing your desire for your partner to gag you and force you to orgasm, your partner is wondering how to best tell you that he really wants to try something new. While your interests may not line up exactly, putting them out in the open allows each of you the opportunity to get what you most need.

If you do decide to take that chance, open up and share your fantasies with someone else, it's ideal to do so in a safe, supportive environment—which means doing more than talking. It means having a conversation.

The art of conversation is something that's nearly lost in today's modern world of texts, multitasking, and emoticons. While almost anyone can talk, many people don't know how to have a real conversation. A conversation involves two (or more) people interacting with each other in an open, honest, respectful, supportive way. That sounds nice, but what does it even mean?

First, it means when you're the speaker, you get the chance to say what you want and need to say without being interrupted, judged or rushed. However, you also have the responsibility of not hogging the conversation; it's a dialogue, not a monologue.

When you are the listener, your job is just to listen and absorb. Nothing more. Don't wait impatiently for the speaker to finish so that you can say the thing that's been on the tip of your tongue for five minutes. Don't interject, interrupt or make frowny faces at the other person. When the other person is finished, think about what he or she has said, and then respond. As the listener, it's also your responsibility to help create a safe space for the speaker by not cutting him off, getting defensive or dismissing his opinion. Be mindful of your own triggers—those topics that make you uncomfortable or uneasy—and try to approach those topics in particular calmly and carefully.

Huh. Turns out, a good sexual conversation sounds an awful lot like therapy, doesn't it? And in many ways it is: a place to explore important, sometimes difficult, issues with someone who cares about you and your well-being. The end goal is to arrive at a place of supportive understanding (and then to go off and have great sex with your conversation partner, which is one way it's different from therapy, at least for most people).

If you're already in a relationship where you're comfortable talking about and exploring your fantasies together, then you're in the perfect place to start stretching your boundaries and comfort zones and really getting down to dirty business.

No matter who you're talking to, don't forget that one of the most important parts of any sex conversation is safety. In fact, it's so important that the entire next chapter is devoted to it. Don't take the next step on your kinky adventure until you talk about limits, safewords and setting boundaries. (See Chapter Three: Yes, No and Maybe: Consent and More, for more information on this aspect of communication.)

Just as I've never regretted having a safe sex conversation with a partner or potential partner, I've never regretted having the "I'm kinky and this is what I like. What do you like?" conversation with a partner. Having an open, honest conversation is the first step to building a strong sexual foundation, one that will hold you up even during the most rough-and-tumble kinky play.

Get Your Passport Stamped: Start a Dialogue

1. Make Sex Jars

Write down twenty-five (or fifty, or who knows, even one hundred) kinky things you're interested in or curious about on strips of paper or index cards, and put them into a jar or container. Have your partner do the same (in a different jar). Each night, take one slip from your partner's jar and read it aloud. Have your partner read one of yours aloud in return. You don't have to talk about what you read or take any actions. This is a great, safe way to start exploring kink in a low-pressure environment.

2. Use Nonverbal Cues

Sometimes having an actual conversation—one person talking, the other person listening and responding—isn't an option. Perhaps, like many of us, you clam up when it comes time for you to speak your mind. Or perhaps you're in a long-distance relationship and your predilection for hairbrush spanking isn't something you want to discuss over video chat.

That's when it's time to break out pen and paper, use body language, do an online quiz together, share your favorite fetish photos or share other nonverbal clues of your personal likes and dislikes. You could even go through the Fetishes and Interests section of the Glossary on page 167, and mark the ones that interest you. Another option is to visit a site like fetlife.com, which has a huge list of fetishes to choose from. If you and your partner happen to share one or more, that's a great place to begin.

3. Read Together

One of the best, safest ways to start exploring your kinks together is to read sexy stuff out loud to each other. Try picking up an erotic anthology, and then choosing a story at random (or have your partner choose a story that he or she would like you to read aloud). Once you're done reading, talk about the story together, making things as personal or impersonal as you feel comfortable with. Sometimes talking about a fetish or fantasy in the context of fiction allows everyone to feel more open, and you'll be surprised at what you can learn about your partner, or even yourself.

4. Go to the Toy Store

If you have a good sex toy store in your area, suggest an outing with your partner. There, you'll find vibrators, handcuffs, dildos, ball gags, riding crops, fake vaginas, velvet corsets, butt plugs…the list is endless. Wandering around a sex toy store gives you both a chance to check things out in a playful, nonthreatening manner outside your usual sex places.

While you're there, keep an eye on what your partner shows an interest in. Does he have his eye on that leather slapper in the corner, or did he head straight for the nipple clamps? And don't be afraid to point out how much you like the hot-pink vibrator or ask questions about how things work or what they're for—if your partner doesn't know the answer, it gives you the perfect excuse to learn about it together.

5. Get a Tune-Up

That first conversation you have with your partner isn't the be-all and end-all of your kinky sex life. You change. Your partner changes. Every six months or so, have a follow-up conversation to see where you're at. Is there anything that you're no longer interested in? Are there new kinks that you can't wait to try? Something you did once and would like to try again? Follow-up conversations are a great way to check in with each other and renew your commitment to hot, kinky sex.

OPEN YOUR MOUTH:

Shanna Katz on Good Communication

Shanna Katz, M.Ed, ACS, is a Board-Certified Sexologist, sexuality educator and workshop presenter.

In your work as a sex coach and relationship counselor, what do you feel is the biggest impediment to people communicating about their kinky side? How can they overcome this?

I think there is still a lot of stigma around the concept of "kink" in our society, despite there being so much kink-related stuff for public consumption (handcuff jewelry, Rihanna's S/M song, collars as fashion). Because of the stigma, there is a lot of fear around the idea of bringing up one's interesting in kink to partners; what if they reject you, what if they laugh at you, what if they think there is something wrong with you? That being said, kink is so much in the eye of the beholder. I've met couples that think being sexual with the lights on is kinky, while other couples incorporate bondage and power play into their sexual activities, but don't identify as kinky because they don't play in public. Rather than communicate about being kinky, sometimes talking about what might turn you on, or seems sexually interesting to you, might go over better than just saying "I'm kinky" and trying to figure it out from there.

What tips do you have for people who are struggling to accept their own kinky side?

Being kinky is 100 percent okay. Being not kinky is 100 percent okay. However your sexuality looks is 100 percent okay (barring anything not consensual/anyone who cannot consent). If you are turned on by something like power play, spanking, leather, bondage, stockings or exhibitionism, that is fine too. It doesn't mean there is anything wrong with you; to the contrary! You are listening to your body and your mind, and supporting yourself by exploring the things that get your motor going. There is no right way to be turned on, no right way to be sexual. Embrace what works for you, and you will be much more sexually satisfied than people who haven't spent the time and energy to figure out what really works for them (and their partner/s).

Telling your partner that you're kinky or polyamorous or [fill in the blank here with your particular desire or interest] is difficult—and with good reason. It's a dangerous place, with a lot at stake. What tips do you have for opening those lines of communication with your partner?

Sharing a part of yourself can be very scary, especially when it comes to sexuality and there is a possibility of rejection. I'd start slow, and maybe bring up the topic in conversation; ask them if they have seen *Secretary*, or what they think of your friends who have an open relationship. Feel out where your partner is on these topics, and maybe take the time to educate her on the subject. (Leaving *Opening Up* or *Playing Well With Others* on the counter or coffee table might help.)

Once you have a good idea of how they will react, then you can figure out the best way to discuss it. Ideas include writing them a letter, having a face-to-face conversation, or giving them a copy of *When Someone You Love Is Kinky* and asking them to read it over and share their thoughts. Remember that they will need time to digest what you've shared with them, just like you may have needed time to come to this conclusion yourself. Don't pressure them to respond right away, and don't share this information during a super busy time, during sex, or in the middle of a fight. You want it to be calm, and for them to have time to process. May sure they know they can ask questions, and you can explore together. (Sites like NewToKink.com are great for videos on new activities that might seem overwhelming, and concepts like negotiation and aftercare.)

On the other side of that, if your partner comes to you and tells you about his desires, what can you do to support him?

First of all, let your partners know that you hear them, you love them and you support them. It might not seem like that big of a deal to actually say those things, but to individuals struggling about sharing their desires and potentially having a fear of rejection, hearing these things can be a huge weight off their shoulders. Then, continue the conversation. It's nice for you to tell them you are okay with it; it's even better if you ask for some more information, suggestions of books or sites to check out, or inquire as to what you can do as a partner to support his or her journey. Also, make sure that you are able to share some of your desires; relationships are not a one-way street.

What are some tips for staying emotionally healthy and safe while exploring the BDSM world?

Communication, communication, communication. Not only that, but make sure you are explicit and spell things out. If you say "I'm cool with this, but we need to be safe about it," that could mean a lot of things. Instead, say what being "safe" means to you. Is it only playing with each other? Is it getting training on different toys/implements before you use them? Is it checking in every ten minutes to make sure you are both okay? Make sure you both contribute to these definitions so that everyone feels as validated and comfortable with the rules/guidelines/boundaries as possible. Check in regularly, not only after playing/during aftercare, but outside of BDSM spaces/play-time as well. Even if you are both happy as clams, it is good for you to both hear that...and it also sets up a space for one or both of you to bring up concerns or issues without having to wait until something big happens.

What question has no one ever asked you on this topic, but you wish someone would?

What happens if we are kinky/start being kinky...and one day, one of us just isn't as into it anymore?

What's the answer to that question?

This happens SO MUCH. Either two kinky people meet in the BDSM community, start a relationship and then a few months or even years down the road, one of them just isn't as kinky as she or he used to be (or is kinky in different ways), or a couple becomes kinky together, and then eventually, it just isn't as interesting or exciting to one person. There are lots of answers, depending on your relationship. The less kinky person could suggest the kinkier person take on a kinky play partner to satisfy her kinky needs, while maintaining the primary relationship in a less kinky or not kinky way. The two could decide to explore a different or new kink to see if it is a good fit for them both. The kinkier person could initiate having not kinky or less kinky sex, and explore new types of not-kinky sex to figure out what works for them both. The list goes on...but what is important to remember is that people change, and our sexualities change. Just because someone isn't as kinky as he used to be, or is kinky in a new direction, doesn't mean that there is anything wrong with him, or the relationship. It's just part of the journey that we are all on throughout our lives.

JUMP OR FALL? (EXCERPT)

Janine Ashbless

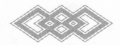

Blayne, what's wrong?"

"Nothing."

"Have I pissed you off? Talk to me!"

"Izzy, please just forget it…" He can't meet my eyes, and his face is all pinched.

"Are you married? Gay?" I'm dead certain he's not gay, not judging by the way he's been watching me since we met. So certain in fact, that I reach out and grab the front of his loose trousers—and it's a good thing he has a hard-on because otherwise that would've been really embarrassing. He jumps when I grasp what is definitely a stiffened cock, and a substantial one at that. "You are so *not* gay," I whisper, rather shocked at myself.

He could shove me off with one push, but instead he plucks my hand from his crotch and folds it against his chest, cradling it. His other hand takes hold of my shoulder. "Izzy, please."

"Have you got a wife then?" He doesn't wear a ring and I've never seen him with a woman, not once in months. He hasn't told me anything. "A girlfriend?"

"No."

"Then what's wrong?"

"Izzy, I really like you."

Oh god: the poverty of the English language, where *I really like you* has to stand in place for everything from *I'm in love* to *I want to fuck your brains out* to *I want you to piss off and leave me alone.*

"Then what's wrong?"

"I really like you," he repeats. "I think you're brilliant, and lovely, and great to work with, and what we've got going here is something so good. I don't want to lose that. I want us to be able to carry on together."

"Like I don't?"

"It won't work."

"I know something that thinks it will." I've already burned my bridges. "This big hard cock of yours thinks we'll do just fine together." I press against him to make my point, and he certainly makes his, right in the wall of my belly. My cunt flutters greedily. He shifts his hips, his eyes darkening. He's holding my hand really tight.

"Believe me," he says hoarsely, "it'll not work out right between us."

"Based on what?"

"Experience."

"Then just fuck me," I whisper. "I'm a big girl, you know: I can handle a one-night stand without going off the rails." I'm not playing fair either, pulling his hand from my bare shoulder down to cup the orb of my breast. He thumbs my nipple instinctively, sending electric flashes through my skin, and I moan.

"Izzy..." He sounds desperate, but he doesn't break. There's something weird going on here.

"Are you scared you'll hurt me?"

Something flickers in his eyes. "Far from it."

"Then what's the problem?"

He drags his hand from my tit and secures both of mine against his chest where I can't do anything naughty with them. I lean into him instead, my thighs burning against his. "Izzy, I have this thing..."

"I know. I can feel it."

He grins without any amusement. "There's this thing I do. It's...a part of my life. It doesn't come as an optional extra. And it's not something you'd be at all happy with."

"What?" For the first time doubt seeps in. "This is a sex thing, is it?"

"Yeah."

"Oh god. Is it something illegal?"

He shakes his head. "No—consenting human adults only. I promise."

"But you think I'll freak out?"

"It's...difficult to understand."

"So you're kinky." I swallow, trying to be blasé. "I can handle that. I'm not a prude."

He pulls a face: disbelief.

"What is it? You like to wear women's underwear? Lick feet? Ah—it's not nappies is it?"

He laughs and then shakes his head.

"Then what? What's so bad I won't even be able to work with you?"

"Can't we just leave it?"

"Too late for that."

He shuts his eyes for a moment. I feel something in the twitch of his muscles. I recognize it: the moment you decide to jump. "You ever been spanked, Izzy?"

"Oh," I say, all sorts of pieces sliding 'round in my mind, trying to find places to fit. "My first boyfriend—I sort of asked him to spank my bottom." To my own surprise I blush. "He called me a freak, and dumped me the next day."

"Ow." For a moment he's smiling again.

"Does that count then?"

"Um. It probably counts as a try."

"So…?"

"So: I'm into pain. In a big way."

"You want me to spank you?"

"Not receiving it. Inflicting it."

"Oh," I say again, wit deserting me. I've got enough sense left to realize that he's talking about more than a bit of playful ass-slapping. "Whoa. You get off on hurting people?"

"Women. Yes." He watches me wince.

"Don't you…" I struggle to frame the question without sounding like a *Daily Mail* editorial. "Doesn't that worry you?"

"Worry me? Yes: all the time. I'm not a psycho, Izzy, or a wife-beater. I'm well aware of the responsibility."

For a long moment there's silence, while I stare at him and try to understand. Because it's still Blayne holding my hands there. He hasn't turned into some weird stranger. It's still Blayne with the anguished eyes and the twisted, rueful mouth, looking so good I want to eat him up. He doesn't have a moustache to twirl or mirror shades or a bloodstained hockey mask. He's the most grounded guy I've met. He doesn't lose his temper when frustrated or throw arty strops, even under provocation. He's the pinup boy for self-control.

Oh. Maybe that does make sense, in a way. And we're getting used to people admitting that they like being caned for kicks. I suppose for everyone who gets off on being whipped there has to be someone who wants to do the whipping. For every bottom there must be a top.

My lips are dry and I run my tongue around to moisten them. "You want to spank me, then, do you?"

He jerks his chin. "Oh yes: I'd like to spank you. I'd like to put you over my knees and pull down your panties and spank your beautiful ass."

Oh god. Oh god. Where is this going? Why aren't I walking away right now? "Hard?"

He sighs. "Gently at first, until your cheeks glow pink. Then harder, as you warm up. I want to see you wriggle. I want to stroke your pussy and make you wet, so wet you're dripping on my hand and my legs, and then I want to spank you right there on your open pussy and make you squeal. I want to make you thrash about, and have to hold you down, and I want to keep going through your wildest struggles. I want to hear you sob and see your mascara streaked down your face with your tears. Do you get it now, Izzy?"

"Oh god."

I get it now. I'm leaning up against this man while he holds my hands so I can't stop him doing anything, and I'm hearing him tell me in a low dreamy voice exactly why I should be scared of him.

And now that he's started, there's no stopping him. A steely look creeps into his eyes: he's seeing himself without flinching and showing me too. "I want to rope you up and slap your pussy and your tits, Izzy. I want to whip you. I want to pinch your nipples until you beg me for mercy. I want to hold you close and see the fear in your eyes and smell the sweat of your pain, and I want to know you trust me to take you through that clear to the other side."

He hesitates, a hitch in his throat.

"I want to be there when all the barriers go down, Izzy, when there's no faking or trying, just your raw naked need. I want to make you come over and over without being able to control yourself, in the middle of everything you dread. I want to inflict unbearable delight. I want to take you places you don't dare go to on your own, and I want to carry you through the dark and hold you and comfort you and kiss the tears away and make you whole again."

He lets go of my hands. There's a bleak and haunted look to him as he sets me on my feet, like a man saying good-bye.

"So now you know."

"Shit."

"Yeah."

How do you react when someone you love tells you he wants to hurt you? That he gets pleasure from your pain? We don't like those kinds of people, do we? We hate and fear them. Since I was little I had, like most girls, run away from hurt. We don't get into fights, we don't ride our bikes down steps just to see what happens, we don't skin our knees and get up and keep going.

"Okay," I admit. "That scares the hell out of me."

He nods. *Told you so.*

I put my hand on the wall, because my legs feel wobbly and my body's quivering. I want to feel something solid to lean on. The painted bricks are cold on my bare shoulder. Blayne turns as I do, so we're face-to-face, still close as lovers. It's the intimacy of confession. "It turns me on too," I whisper.

His eyes widen slightly, but what I read there is doubt and concern. He lifts his hand to my face and traces his fingers down my cheek.

"Just listening to you talk makes me…" I swallow hard. "Wet. I'm all wet." My knickers are sodden, my pussy swollen and heavy. But, amazingly, he shakes his head.

"I'm not trying to convert you, Izzy. It's something you either get or you don't."

"I do get it. I think. A bit. The pain thing…" I'm trying to think past the tender, regretful caress of his fingers. "When I had my tattoo done, it was horrible for the first five minutes. I had to force myself to stay put. And then this endorphin rush kicked in I guess—and forty minutes later it was still hurting but I just wanted it never to stop. Pain's...a weird thing."

"Complicated," he agrees. "More so than we're ever told." He smiles. "I didn't even know you had a tattoo."

"Want to see it?"

He nods. "Please." I think I glimpse then how vulnerable he is in his need, and how isolated. How he must hold himself on the edge, waiting permission to jump. I turn my face to the wall, pulling up the clingy cotton of my top to expose my lower spine and slipping the top button of my trousers to drop them low on my hips. It's a barbed tribal-style tattoo at the small of my back, nothing very original I suppose, but I love it. The delta of black thorns is like a magical ward over the cleft of my bum.

Blayne touches the ink, and I shiver all over. Then he slides to his knees behind me. I feel the first touch of his lips and I'm flying, my heart pounding in my chest, my head full of the beat of wings. The tip of his tongue follows, warm and moist, tracing the path of the tattoo. I hear his soft groan. My fingers feel clumsy, but I manage to slip three more fly buttons and here is cool air on my cheeks as my trousers fall away to expose the curves of my out-thrust rear.

He can't resist that, can he? My bottom, offered to him as a gift, tied in the lace ribbons of my very tiny thong?

No, he can't resist.

His hands cover the twin globes of my ass, warm on my cool flesh. Then with a surge he's standing again, pressing into me from behind, squashing my breasts to the brick wall and grinding into me with a cock so hard and imperious that he seems likely to split the fabric of his own pants. He grips the rope of my braid and slowly tugs my head back, and with the other hand he delves under the jut of my ass, between my thighs, scrabbling aside the elasticized lace of my gusset. Finding wet. So much wet.

"You weren't lying, were you?" he breathes in my ear.

I whimper, words fleeing as he explores every whorl and hollow and swell of my sex. Blayne growls under his breath, a bass line to the soft high noises I'm making.

CHAPTER THREE

YES, NO AND MAYBE: CONSENT AND MORE

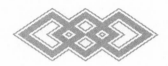

> *...I thought well as well him as another and then I asked him with my eyes to ask again yes and then he asked me would I yes to say yes my mountain flower and first I put my arms around him yes and drew him down to me so he could feel my breasts all perfume yes and his heart was going like mad and yes I said yes I will Yes.*
>
> —*Ulysses*, James Joyce

If there is anything more full of consent than Molly Bloom's soliloquy in James Joyce's novel, *Ulysses*, I don't know what it is. In fact, for years, I've said I want to get this entire soliloquy tattooed on some part of my body as a reminder of what joyous, excited, informed consent can look like. (Of course, that single sentence is more than 4,300 words, so I'd have to find a fairly big body part in order to fit it properly.)

In the kinky community, *consent* means that you are saying yes to a shared experience. Typically you do this by providing explicit, informed verbal agreement. (I'll break down some of those words in just a bit.) In other words, by saying, clearly and with no uncertainty: Yes.

But what about all the rest? Do you need a safeword? A contract? Some kind of complicated verbal agreement? A secret handshake?

Yes and no.

My first kinky partner and I had a very specific but simple way of asking for and giving consent.

"Do you like that?"

"Yes."

"Do you want more?

"Yes."

"Can we try this?"

"Yes."

I didn't even really know that we were what others would call kinky, that we were doing something that could be considered outside the "norm" or that we were supposed to have some kind of consent process. It was pre-Internet, so we couldn't just go and Google what we were supposed to be doing. Our foray into kink was mostly an outgrowth of being young and in lust and just having tons and tons of sex. It wasn't as though there was a line we suddenly stepped over and we were in BDSM land. We were just exploring, and we instinctively understood that what we were doing required both of us to want it and to agree to it. If one of us asked a question and the answer was anything but yes—no, maybe, I'm not sure, what do you mean?—we stopped and talked about it before we did it.

My early experience is unusual, I'm sure, and probably some people who hear that story will wrinkle their noses at it. We didn't have a safeword. We didn't set boundaries ahead of time. We didn't have a formal contract or a secret handshake. We certainly didn't have informed consent (informed, meaning that we understood the risks of what we were about to undertake and agreed to them). We just had open, honest communication, and it worked for us at the time.

Since then, I've had partners with whom I've needed something more spelled out. And other potential partners that didn't become partners because we couldn't find a way to set boundaries together.

Getting and giving consent will likely vary from person to person and relationship to relationship, and even from moment to moment within a specific sexual encounter.

However, two elements always stay the same:

1. Consent is probably the most important element of any sexual activity, whether you're kinky or not (it holds top honors with safety, and the two often go hand in hand).

2. There is no single right way to get and give consent or to create boundaries. All you really need is a way to say yes—and perhaps more importantly, no—to the person (or people) you're about to interact with.

That's the simple side of it. But not surprisingly, consent is a complicated topic. Within the concept of consent, we're actually talking about a whole lot of important ideas all wrapped up in one big gift-wrapped package.

One important concept in that package is the one that says that true consent must be *explicit*. Saying nothing is not giving consent. Saying no is not giving consent (except in the case where this is a kink that you're interested in exploring with an experienced, trustworthy partner and you've worked it out ahead of time). The only way to give consent is to state it, either in a contract, a verbal agreement or some other clear and unequivocal way.

Within the BDSM community, there are a number of philosophies around the idea of giving consent and setting boundaries. Perhaps the oldest code is one of "Safe, Sane and Consensual" (SSC), which means that the participants engage in safe activities, that everyone involved is in a sane state of mind and that everyone has explicitly consented.

A newer tenet, and one that's gained popularity, is "Risk Aware Consensual Kink," often called RACK for short. The concept behind it is that all sex—including all kinky sex—has inherent risks, and that any individual who's engaging in BDSM play is informed of what those risks are, has some knowledge and understanding of how to mitigate them and is agreeing to participate with those risks in mind. Essentially, this philosophy puts the onus on individuals to evaluate risks versus rewards for themselves.

In the end, the definitions and acronyms don't matter as much as you knowing your own mind, expressing your own limits and listening when others express theirs, and feeling comfortable that whoever you're playing with will be respectful of everyone's choices.

A good way to think about it might be to imagine BDSM as an extreme sport like mountain climbing. There are always risks, but the differences in risks between using an interior climbing wall with a harness under the supervision of a coach and summiting a tall mountain with a novice climber are great, and both experiences can be made safer with proper training, communication and equipment.

So it is with sex. Every time you have sex of any sort, you run the risk of catching an STD or being injured (emotionally or physically). But some sexual activities have a higher risk of injury than others. Spanking, for example, is relatively safe, provided that you understand where and how to hit someone without causing injury. Something like knife play, where the skin is actually broken open, is more dangerous, and there are types of play, such as breath play, that are considered so risky that many people in the BDSM community stay away from them entirely.

So, when it comes to knowing the risks and saying yes anyway, it's best to never assume and never guess. And never, ever agree to something that you don't want. Consent is a dance: one person asks, one person answers. Even in a group activity, each person should have a chance to ask and answer, to call and respond.

When you're the one asking for consent, it means that you are clearly engaging and listening to your partner's needs, and that you understand what you're asking of your partner. When you're the one giving consent, you're making it clear that you are ready to begin, and that you understand and are saying yes to what your partner is asking of you, without reservation.

Saying yes is also what provides the fine, but firm, line between kinky sex and abuse or violence. In fact, when it comes to the law in some areas of the world, informed consent could be the *only* thing that protects you and your partner(s) from abuse charges—and sometimes even that is not enough (see more on this in Chapter Seven: Staying Safe, page 121).

Not all of this negotiation happens at the beginning of an experience. Typically, play is structured so that at any point, any of the partners can change their mind and withdraw their consent. Saying things like "thank you," or "may I have another?" aren't just sexy pillow talk; they also let your partner know that you're fine to continue playing. A good partner will pay attention to your breathing and tone when you speak, and can learn a lot from what you say and how you say it.

This is also where safewords or safe symbols are used as an explicit way of removing consent.

Safewords can be anything that you can say quickly and easily in the heat of the moment, and that neither you nor your partner will forget. Some people like to use simple, common words like *stop* or *no* but those can be tricky because they're also sometimes used during consensual coercion play. Colors can be one good option, with *green* meaning "good," *yellow* meaning "I need to slow down" or "I'm starting to feel uncomfortable" and *red* meaning "stop." Another good choice for a word is something that has a special meaning to you and your current partners, that isn't easy to mishear or misinterpret and that you would likely never say in the normal course of sex. Whenever possible, try not to choose words that are homonyms, because during sex, your partner won't be able to tell the different between *bear* (meaning "stop") and *bare* (meaning something else entirely). Personally, I prefer short, simple words that are easy to say, understand and remember, but I know people whose safewords are vegetables (*asparagus*), animals (*triceratops*), and the name of the restaurant where they had their first date.

Safe symbols are actions or responses that can be taken when one partner has had enough, such as dropping a teddy bear, squeezing a hand or ringing a bell. Often used when speech is restricted, safe symbols can also be incorporated into a scene as a sexy prop; in a Daddy/daughter scene, for example, having the "daughter" hold a teddy bear gives the sign that play is fine to continue. As soon as the toy gets dropped, it's a sign that play is over.

Get Your Passport Stamped: Yes You Said Yes You Will Yes

1. Make a Yes-Maybe-No List.
This list will be primarily for you, but is also something that you can share with a partner in the future. Find a list of kinky interests (use the list at the back of this book on page 167, do an online search for BDSM, or check out a site like fetlife.com for their long list of fetishes) and start building your list of things you want to try, things you're curious about and things that you are sure you don't want. Start with broad strokes—bondage, spanking, domination—and then narrow in as far as you can. If you like spanking, do you like to be bare-

bottomed? Do you like a hand or a paddle or both? Do you get off on the pain of it, the lack of power, the marks that a spanking can leave afterward, or does it vary from time to time? Does the thought of having someone put her hand around your neck turn you on or freak you out?

The more you know about your own boundaries, the more you can teach your partner and the better advocate you will be for your own boundaries. For example, I know that one thing I absolutely cannot stand is to be tickled. But it isn't just that I don't care for it; it's that I know myself well enough to know that I can't control my movements if someone's tickling me (or even about to do so). I kick, punch, flail and do anything possible to get out of the situation and that puts both myself and my partner in danger.

2. Practice Saying No (and Yes)
Saying no can be hard. Saying no to someone we love, lust after, respect or just want to play with can be especially hard. But if you're a submissive or a bottom (or taking on that type of role in any way), it's your responsibility to say no when you need to say no. No one else can do it for you. No matter how attentive a top/dom/partner is, the only way he or she can know for sure that you've had enough is if you say so.

If you're someone who has trouble saying no in your life, try it outside of the bedroom for a bit first. Politely turn down that invitation you didn't have time for. Say no to the telemarketer. Get used to creating boundaries outside the bedroom, and then slowly move your "no" into your sex life.

If, on the other hand, you're someone who has trouble saying yes to your own needs, create a space where you can do just that. If your partner is willing, give him or her a list of things you'd like to do. Be explicit. Don't write, *I'd like to be spanked,* because that doesn't give your partner a good guide. Instead write, *I'd like to be laid across your lap with my panties down while you lightly spank my ass with your bare hand.*

Then set up a play session where your partner asks you if you'd like to do each of the things on that list. Each time he asks something you'd like, say yes, loudly and clearly. Spend a little time savoring each delicious reward of your clear consent before you go on to the next item on your list.

3. Ask Your Questions Clearly

There's another side to this too: if you like to be the more dominant partner, learn how to ask questions that give you the answers you need. Ask a specific question each time you do something new. Questions like "Do you like it when I touch you here?" and "Would you like me to do that again?" give your partner a chance to answer with a simple yes or no. Open-ended questions provide more details, but can be harder for someone to answer. "What would you like me to do to you?" or "How would you like me to spank you?" might be too open-ended for some people who are in the midst of sexual pleasure, so you could try a question that gives options like, "Do you prefer me to spank you with my bare hand or should I get out that new paddle we bought?" Whatever you ask, if you are unsure of the answer, ask again. Turn it into play. To my mind, there's nothing sexier than someone laying out my options for me, and promising that one of them is going to happen. All I have to do is say yes.

KNIT ONE AND TIE ME UP, TOO

Kristina Wright

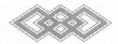

I hate winter. I hate the cold, I hate the snow, I hate the clothes. Everyone is bundled up in ten different layers of clothing and wherever you go, the heat is cranked up so you have to strip off half of those layers and lug them around with you. I even hate the hobbies of winter—skiing, ice-skating and, when the weather is too cold to even venture outside, knitting. Knitting is the most ridiculous, frustrating, pointless venture I can imagine. You take a ball of overpriced yarn and two needles and proceed to make a substandard version of something you could buy for half the price at a department store. I just don't get it. Of course, I can't knit, so what do I know?

My girlfriend, Becca, however, is a little knitting demon. She knits sweaters, she knits socks, she knits mittens and tea cozies (for her grandmother) and hats and scarves. She knitted a blanket and pillow shams for our couch and a cover for our dog Brody's bed. Becca doesn't just like knitting, she loves it. It is her passion and she knits year-round, but in the winter she turns into one of Santa's elves with her knitting needles click-clicking away late into the night, night after night. Sometimes I think I hear those knitting needles in my sleep, only to wake up and find out I wasn't dreaming, she's actually knitting in bed next to me.

Despite her questionable taste in hobbies, I adore my Becca. She's a girl's girl and doesn't have a mean bone in her body. So when she said to me one night, all sweetness and smiles, "Would you help me roll my yarn?" I tried very hard not to roll my eyes and said I would, even though I would have rather kept reading my mystery novel.

We were lying in bed, Becca in her flannel pajamas and socks (that she knit herself, of course) and me in just a T-shirt and shorts. I think part of the reason Becca knits is because she has such a cold-blooded nature. She's always cold and always trying to warm up. She handed me a skein of suede-soft, orangey-red yarn and told me to roll it into a ball. She began doing the same with another skein of the same color.

I stifled a sigh and began rolling. Still, I couldn't help asking, "Why do you bother doing this?" The whole thing seemed pointless to me.

Rolling her skein at twice the pace I was, Becca said, "To keep it from knotting up. If the yarn is snarled somewhere in the center of the skein, I'll have to cut it. This way, the yarn stays unknotted and perfect."

"Oh." It was a perfectly logical reason, but it still annoyed the crap out of me. "This is a pretty color. What are you going to make?"

"A blindfold to go with the bondage straps I already made."

My yarn-rolling abilities ceased right there. "Uh...what?"

Becca kept her eyes demurely on her yarn. "I figured I'd make something you'd truly appreciate."

Not only had I lost all manual dexterity, I also seemed to have lost the power of speech. "Um...huh?"

Becca laughed. "Look at the bedposts."

I looked. I don't know why I hadn't noticed them before, but sure enough, hanging from each of the mahogany bedposts was a thin orangey-red strap. I would have called them scarves, despite their narrow width, if Becca hadn't told me what they were. "And you're going to make what?"

"A blindfold," she said, showing infinite patience for her girlfriend that had just become a blathering fool. "I think it'll enhance the experience."

"Uh, I see." This was all new to me. Becca was great in bed and we'd enjoyed more than our share of hot, wild sex, but bondage was something she'd never so much as hinted at wanting to try. "So, who's tying up whom, exactly?"

"Well, I thought you might want to tie me up," she said. She wasn't looking at me, but there was no mistaking the quiver of nervous excitement in her voice and the blush in her cheeks.

"You're blushing the same color as your yarn."

She giggled. "And you're getting that rough, gravelly voice you get when you're thinking about throwing me down and fucking me."

"Am I?"

"You are."

"Hmm," I murmured. "Maybe I need to stop thinking about it and do it."

I expected Becca to protest a little or at least insist we finish rolling her yarn. Instead, she tossed her neatly rolled ball of yarn and my half-rolled skein into the bag at the end of the bed. Then she looked at me expectantly.

"Anxious, huh?" I couldn't help but smile. "Okay, so now what?"

"Whatever you want," she said, a little breathlessly.

I pretended to think about that for a minute, though I already knew what I wanted. "Maybe you should get naked."

"Good idea."

She started with the buttons on her pajama top. With deliberate slowness, she slipped each button free. Finally, all the buttons were undone and her top hung open, giving me just the merest glimpse of the curve of her breasts. It made me want more. A lot more.

"Take off the pants," I said.

She knelt up and hooked her thumbs in the sides of the flannel pants. She peeled them down until they were bunched around her knees. Then, she sat down with a grace I'd never possess and pulled them off. In the process, her shirt opened up, displaying one hard, rosy nipple.

"Take off the top, too." I wanted her naked. Naked and tied to the bed. Just the thought made me wet. "Quickly."

As if sensing my impatience, she didn't try to tease me. The top fluttered to the ground with the bottoms and Becca sat on the bed in her pink panties and pink knitted socks.

"Socks," I said.

She made an impatient sound. "My feet are cold. I want to keep them on."

"Fine. Lie down," I said.

"What about my panties?"

"They stay on."

I don't know if it was the thought of what I might do to her or the tone of my voice, but Becca made a sweet little noise and said, "Okay."

She stretched out on the bed, arms overhead. I got up and went to the head of the bed, tying the knitted strap she had already secured to the bedpost around her right wrist. "Nice," I said, giving the strap a little tug. "Soft, but sturdy."

Becca giggled again. "I thought so."

I moved to her right ankle and did the same. Pretty soon, I had

Becca tied down and spread out before me. She looked incredible and I stood there for several long moments, just watching her.

She began to squirm under my gaze. "Well? Aren't you going to do something?"

"Hush," I said, softly but firmly. "I like looking at you this way."

She sighed and wiggled, watching me watch her. But she didn't say anything.

What I didn't tell her was that I was as anxious as she was. I knelt between her spread legs, staring at her panty-covered crotch. "Are you wet?"

She raised her hips as much as the straps would allow. "Why don't you find out?"

I inhaled deeply. I could smell her. "You're wet."

She nearly growled in frustration. "Are you going to touch me?"

I laughed. "Maybe. If you're nice."

Becca looked at me. "Oh, I'm nice. I'm very, very nice. Touch me. Please?"

I held my hand over her cunt, not touching her. Slowly, as slowly as she'd taken off her pajamas, I used one finger to trace the edge of her panties. Up the inside of one thigh, then along the top, from hip bone to hip bone, then down the other thigh. I was careful not to touch her skin or to press too hard, using only my fingertip on the hot pink satin trim of her panties.

Becca squirmed and panted under my gentle touch, trying to maneuver so I would touch more. "You're making me crazy," she said, her voice heavy with a mixture of arousal and annoyance. "Touch me."

I smacked the inside of her thigh and she gasped, more from the surprise of the contact than any real pain. "I'm in charge, remember?"

"Yes, Ma'am," she breathed.

"Good girl."

If I'd had more self-control, I would have continued teasing Becca for a while, but I wanted to touch her as badly as she wanted to be touched. Still, it wouldn't do to give in too much. I knew I could get her off quickly, and myself, too, but I wanted to build the anticipation. For both of us.

I leaned over her, running my fingers along her lips. She kissed my fingertips eagerly. "Suck," I said, sliding my index finger between her lips.

Obediently, Becca sucked. I slid my middle finger into her mouth and she kept sucking. I pulled my fingers free from her mouth and ran my wet fingertips over her nipple. She gasped and arched her back and I did the same to the other nipple. Back and forth, I stroked her pale-pink nipples until they were hard and she was whimpering.

"More," she whispered. "Please."

"More?"

She nodded.

Using both hands, I pinched her nipples. Hard. She moaned, pushing her breasts up to my hands. Her back was arched, her head pressed into the pillow, and her eyes closed so she didn't see what I did next. I leaned over her and sucked first one rigid nipple between my lips, then the other.

"Oh!" she gasped.

I pulled back far enough to look into her half-closed eyes. "More?"

She nodded. "Yes, please."

I moved down until I was kneeling between her legs again. There was a small wet spot on the crotch of her panties. I'd done that. I had done that just by touching and sucking her nipples. I decided I liked being in charge.

I grabbed the insides of her thighs and spread her wider. Then

I leaned down and placed the gentlest of kisses right on her panty-covered cunt. She bucked and moaned as if I'd just slid my entire fist inside her.

"I guess that means more," I said.

Becca just moaned.

I pressed my mouth to her panties, finding the hard ridge of her swollen clit just above the wet spot she'd made. I gently licked her clit through the cotton of her panties until the wet spot had spread and the fabric clung to her.

"Oh god, oh god," she whimpered, shifting her hips against my mouth. "More. God, please, more."

I would have laughed at her desperate tone, but I was thinking the same thing. More. More Becca. Now. I hooked one finger in the leg hole of her panties and pulled them aside, revealing her swollen, wet cunt to my gaze. She arched and gasped at the feeling of my warm breath on her, but I didn't touch her. Not just yet. I marveled at her cunt, swollen and deeper red than I remembered, her clit hard and glistening like a ripe, exotic berry.

"Please," she begged. "Please."

I couldn't deny her. I ran the flat of my tongue over her swollen clit and was rewarded by a wail that would no doubt have the neighbors calling the police. Not that I cared. Again and again, I slowly lapped Becca's clit, knowing the constant licking would drive her mad because it felt so good and yet still wouldn't be quite enough to get her off.

She kept pushing her hips up, pulling hard against the straps that kept her in place. "Faster, more, lick me, lick me, please," she panted. I doubted she had any idea what she was saying.

As I licked her clit, I teased the opening of her pussy with one finger. I heard the bed creak as she strained to push herself closer and, out of fear she'd break the bed, I slid my finger into her. She was so wet, I wasn't sure she could even feel me. I added a second finger and began pushing them in and out of her in the same, slow rhythm I was using to lick her clit.

"Oh, oh, oh," Becca grunted, moving her hips against me at twice the pace I stroked her. "More, please."

I pushed a third finger into her, entwining my fingers as I fucked her with them. I could feel her pulse through her clit, the steady throb-throb as I licked and fucked her. She grunted and moaned, thrashing as much as her bonds would allow, which was more than I expected. I had to use one hand to anchor her hip; she was thrusting so hard against me I thought she'd knock my teeth out with her pelvic bone.

"I need to come," she gasped. "Please."

The bondage might have been a new thing, but I knew what Becca needed to get off. I sucked her clit between my lips and felt her cunt ripple around my fingers. Her swollen flesh throbbed around my hand, pulsing like a wild thing as I sucked her clit, flicking the tip of my tongue across it again and again until her entire body went rigid and she nearly levitated off the bed as she came in my mouth.

I held her clit between my lips as she came, sucking it with unrelenting determination as she moaned and wailed and bucked against me. My fingers were still buried inside her, the muscles of her cunt so tight around me I didn't think she'd ever let me go. Even after her moans faded to soft whimpers, I kept nursing at her clit, gently letting it slide between my lips before reclaiming it.

"Oh, please, I can't take any more," she whispered finally.

Only then did I stop. I looked up at her, grinning like the love-struck fool I was. I hadn't even gotten off yet, but I felt amazingly satisfied. "Wow. That was incredible. I think I'm going to want to tie you up a lot."

"Only if we take turns," she said.

My pulse jumped at the thought. "Hmm…yeah. Maybe next time you'll have that blindfold made."

Becca laughed. "Are you saying you like me knitting now?"

I nuzzled and nipped the inside of her damp thigh. "Oh yeah, babe. Oh hell yeah."

BEARERS

Nikki Magennis

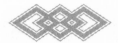

S he's standing there looking, for the first time, I believe, disarmed.
Biting her lip a bit. That full, pretty, rose-red lip. Caught in her
pearl-white teeth. I like it. I like her a little uncertain. She seduced
me already running around like an angelic go-go dancer, but now,
swaying on her heels and picking at her sleeve, she's fucking dyna-
mite.

Yeah. I like Jacqueline like this.

"How about if—?" I make a decision. Step into the shoes of the
person I wish I was. I lean over and kiss Jacqueline, meeting her over
the open takeaway bag, the smell of chicken chow mien and sesame
oil mixing in our mouths as I taste her soft uncertainty, her sharp
want and her sweet pleasure.

She moans a little. I think I feel her melt. And now I know what
to do, what exactly to do.

"Is this okay?" I murmur, as I walk round the table, take her by the hand and pull her to me. "I'm going to strip you, and lick you, and fuck you. Is that all okay?"

"Yes," she says, and her eyes are violet and dark.

"And how about this," I say, not missing a beat. I pull her hands behind her back and circle her wrists with my own hands. She's not a delicate thing, this woman, but I am bigger and I get a rush of feeling like a river must feel when it swallows a stream. "What if I tied you down?"

She nods. Her eyes are like mirrors now, wet and shining. "What else?" I say, half to myself. I bite on my beard, scrape the stubbly hairs with my teeth. "I could put you over my knee."

She laughs, but I see her chest rise and fall, those perfect tits shivering a little.

"I don't know what it is, Jacqueline. You make me want to do stuff."

"Yeah?" she asks.

I shake my head. "You're so fucking lovely, I want to corrupt you," I say, softly.

She dances tighter into my arms. "Say it."

"You want it. All that nasty stuff," I say, into the cup of her collarbone.

"Mmm-hm." she says, and her voice drags across my heart, scrapes over my skin and tugs at the head of my cock.

We practically dragged each other to bed. I barely got my shoes off before we were battling at each other, moths against each other's dim lights, looking for a way in. I found scraps of bare skin under her clothes and grabbed at them. I felt the heat between my fingers, the good solidity of her, how she was lithe and demanding in my hands.

I never did manage to strip her as promised. I had to be inside her, it was that simple. She tore open my trousers and we fumbled with a rubber, hands shaky, barely able to smile. She leaned back against her dressing table and I splayed her legs and held them open.

I planted my cock inside her, dug it in firmly. She responded with a loud "Oh!" as if she'd just remembered something important. And we fucked at light speed.

It was all over in a flash, inevitably. We were overtaken by our bodies, beaten insensible to the finish line by twin orgasms. Crashed into each other, speaking in tongues, my cock weeping into her, her clinging to me and dribbling on my shoulder.

A spectacular, but fairly breathless coupling.

What was unexpected was what happened next. Without moving, Jacqueline opened her mouth and bit me. Hard.

I liked her bite. It made sense. I don't know if that sentence does or if you understand what I'm saying now, but I don't care.

It all made sense. We did.

I turned her 'round and bent her over the dressing table and without saying a word, slapped her arse hard enough to leave a print. I waited long enough for the echo in my head to fade, while I watched her face in the mirror. Her eyes were closed. There was a slight sheen on her upper lip, and a spreading tide of red on her cheek. In the half-light of her bedroom I could smell dust and laundry powder and the sweet apple smell of her sweat.

At last, she moved away. Everything was slower now, like we were moving underwater. She opened a drawer and pulled out some balled-up tights, black nylon. Held them out to me in her fist.

"Do it," she said, raising her brows. "Tie me down."

"To what?"

"I don't care. So long as it's not a moving car."

I caught her wrist.

"Listen. I'll tie you to the bed and maybe slap you a little. If you don't like it, say stop. Okay?"

"Is that a safeword? Stop? Seems pretty…obvious."

"Works for me."

I kept her wrist. Wrapping the leg of a nylon 'round it, I anchored it to the bedpost. Taking her second wrist, I stretched her arm straight and tied the nylon like a cuff. Her left ankle, I held more firmly, tugged at her a little to get her in position. By the time she was spread-eagled, I was hard again and ready to go.

I still had a pair of tights in my hand, weightless, soft and black. I pulled them taut between my hands, lifted them so she could see what I was doing—winding them around my fists and stretching until I had a strong rope.

I brought it down. Lowered it gently, covered her breasts like a bandeau. I pressed down, my hands on either side of her, binding her tightly. Under the nylon her breasts spilled over, and I began squeezing those beautiful tits. Hard. Until she gasped. I bit the nipples and moved down, dragging at her skin, roughing it a little, pulling the nylon over her curves and hollows.

She was whimpering, and I liked that a lot. I stopped and rested the fabric band on her hips, so that it cut over her pubic bone, just at the top of the rust-brown curls of her hair. Now the tights were bisecting her body, and her bottom half was bucking up toward me.

"Please," she said. "Oh god, I want you to lick me."

"It's not up to you," I said quietly.

She kind of forced this humming sound out of her lips, then, because she knew she couldn't say anything to change my mind, but she apparently had to make noise. I listened to her low, tuneless song and then I pulled the tights between her legs, over her mound and up behind her ass. Now I could seesaw them over her clit, tug on one end and make a shiver run over her whole body. I rocked them back and forth a little, watching how she twisted and strained against her ties.

Then I bent down and put my face between her legs and tasted her. Apple and earth. Sharp and sweet. I sipped at her clit. Above me, she sobbed with pleasure, her voice muffled as if she was burying her face in the pillow. I slid my tongue inside her, as deep as I could, and heard her breath stop. One more flick at her clit.

She came like a storm breaking. I think because she was tied down it prolonged it. There was nowhere for the sensation to go, so it rolled around, rippling and waving and repeating. I could feel the pulse of her pussy under my lips, the little spasms.

When I kissed her, afterward, her mouth was as soft as petals.

CHAPTER FOUR

PACKING YOUR TOY BOX

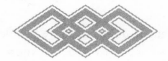

When I was in college, I started reviewing sex toys on a regular basis. Partly because I was broke and the companies sent me the toys for free if I agreed to test them and write a review, but mostly because I wanted to know more about the toys themselves. Sure, I'd been to a few sex toy stores, but back then the stores in my hometown were a little scary and dirty, there were no other women in the places and they mostly stocked movies. I was young and shy and more than a little intimidated, so I wasn't about to start feeling up dust-covered dildos to see which ones I liked best, nor was I going to ask what the black-and-silver chain harness in the corner was supposed to be used for.

Instead, I started getting "discreet" packages delivered to my door. I put *discreet* in quotes because that's what the websites promised, but it only took my postman one trip to look at that unidentified shipping object and give me a sly grin as he handed it over. Eventually, we became friends and he would leave the packages around the corner of the house when I wasn't home, sometimes with a hand-written note about what he guessed was inside. (He was almost never right, by the way, but it was a lot of fun to see what he *thought* he was delivering.)

Since that time, I've reviewed hundreds of sex toys. The experience taught me a lot about the toys themselves—what they're designed to be used for, what they really should be used for (those two aren't always the same), what makes a quality toy and what makes me want to throw something out the window (sorry, poor dude outside minding your own business—I wasn't actually aiming for you with that glitter-filled dildo).

By trying out hundreds of toys, I've also learned a surprising amount about myself and what I like. If you're interested in pain, you can learn just how much pain you like by trying out a bunch of different floggers or nipple clamps. The difference between "Oh yeah, that smarts a little" and "Oh my god, my ass is on fire" shows you just how many choices there are along the pain spectrum.

Sex toys aren't just things that come wrapped in discreet packages from a store, of course. When I say "sex toys," I basically mean anything that can be used by one or more people during play: vibrators, dildos, cuffs, collars, pretty panties, bondage tape, stockings, high heels, masks, a doctor's outfit. Ice, heat, knives, candles, showerheads. Even the pleasure tools that you carry with you all the time—hands, teeth, nails and your brain are some of the most intoxicating toys you can employ. (Check out the Toys and Objects section in the Glossary on page 173 for a sample of all the goodies you can buy, create or use to heighten kinky sex.)

Toys are especially great for solo play and exploration. I recommend trying toys out on yourself before you hand them over to someone else. Sometimes our eyes are bigger than our pain tolerance—a pair of toothy nipple clamps that looked all shiny and exciting in the store might turn out to be far more than we can actually handle. (Of course, it goes without saying that if you're playing with anything even slightly dangerous, make sure you have a spotter, someone who can step in and get you out of any bad situation that might arise.)

And packing your toy box is about more than just toys. Also consider stocking up on condoms, dental dams, and gloves for safety, towels for spills and cleanups and a first aid kit for emergencies (see Chapter Seven: Staying Safe for tips on creating a first aid kit).

Stamp Your Passport: Discover the Joys of Toys

1. Clean out Your Pantry.

Least sexy recommendation ever, right? Wrong. You'll be surprised at what possible sex toys are hidden away in your home. Apron strings, towels and scarves make great impromptu bondage ties or blindfolds; wooden spoons, hairbrushes and rubber spatulas are lovely to slap against an ass; and ice, sandpaper and zesters are all excellent choices for sensation play. Got an exercise machine? Doesn't that bad boy just seem built for a little bondage? What about a jump rope or a Ping-Pong paddle? You get the idea. Keep your lust glasses on and you just might start to see every household object as a potential new toy.

As always, be careful. Toys scavenged from around the house aren't specifically designed for sex play, so always use your best judgment.

2. Play a Role.

Role-playing can be one of the hottest, dirtiest ways to revel in your kinky interests. Whether you want to play a hot doctor who just has to thoroughly check her newest patient, a lost puppy who is looking for the perfect home with a strong owner, or you're interested in playing out your favorite scene from a movie or book that you adore, finding the perfect toys, accessories, outfits and equipment can help get you and your partner in the right frame of mind. Check out the local thrift or costume stores to build your own outfits for cheap—it can be especially fun to hit the stores with your partner and see what the two of you can build. The anticipation of knowing what happens once you get home and put your new outfits on extends the experience into an all-day lust-fest.

3. Put Your Toys Away.
It's important to take good care of your toys with proper maintenance and cleaning, and to have a place to store them. Invest in something beautiful to hold your toys—perhaps a nice blanket chest with a lock or a set of office-style storage boxes in colors that you like. For a long time I kept my toys in a small carry-on suitcase. It rolled from room to room, locked easily and could be slid under the bed so that it was out of sight. Whatever you decide to get for your toys, make sure it's large enough to hold everything, and that it will keep out dust, dirt, the neighbors and any household creatures (pets and children alike) who can't resist chewing on leather or rubber.

TOY STORY:

Sunny Megatron on the Joys of Kinky Toys

Sunny Megatron is a kink and sexuality educator and the host of the sexual health and wellness web series Outside the Box.

You do a lot of sex toy reviews and write-ups. What are a few types of toys that you recommend people start with if they're looking to start exploring their kinky sides?

One of the most awesome things about kink is you don't have to spend a lot of money to get started. Basic wooden clothespins can be used as clamps on the nipples, labia or scrotum. Inexpensive sleeping masks double as blindfolds. Soft, cotton clothesline is perfect for light bondage and things like wooden spoons or hairbrushes are great for impact play. A microfiber mitt designed for car waxing can lessen the blow of an open-handed spank, or it can feel delightful when lightly dragged across the skin. The plastic rod that opens and closes window blinds makes a deliciously wicked cane that delivers quite a sting. With a little ingenuity, most of us can find an arsenal of kinky items right in our own homes.

Household objects that are repurposed for kinky play are usually referred to as *pervertables*. A basic BDSM tool kit can be constructed inexpensively from items found at hardware, dollar and kitchen stores. For people just starting out, I usually recommend they explore with pervertables first to find out what type of play and items they gravitate toward.

In addition to pervertables, you should have a dedicated sex toy or two at your disposal. Things like a wand-style vibrating toy and a dildo or two are a good start.

Is there a type of toy that seems to get a lot of hype, but that doesn't typically live up to people's hopes for it?

Folks new to kink often reach first for the fuzzy handcuffs. Those are the ultimate kinky starter toy, right? Not exactly. They are one of the worst and most uncomfortable bondage items you can buy. Most people figure this out after wearing them only once. The metal digs into the skin, the fuzzy material can produce friction burns and often they squeeze too tightly. Most wearers only end up bruised or cut after a romp with fuzzy handcuffs but some suffer nerve damage. Luckily, they are so uncomfortable people usually figure out they aren't what they are cracked up to be right off the bat and discontinue use before much damage is done.

Ben wa balls are also a source of disappointment for many people. They are great products but most users aren't aware of how they should be used.

Let's talk more about ben wa balls. I've heard toy store owners say that they're selling out of them after their appearance in *50 Shades of Grey*, but that people want to return them because they end up not liking them. What should people know about them before they buy?

Ben wa balls only cause immediate sexual arousal in a small percentage of women. Anastasia Steele's reaction was not at all typical and was definitely exaggerated to make the scene in the book hotter. Most women can barely detect the vaginal jiggling the balls make when worn. To a lot of us it sort of feels like wearing a tampon. Not at all sexy.

Ben wa balls absolutely can help you have earth-shattering orgasms but not in the way you have been led to think. These products are Kegel muscle exercisers. They are tools to help you strengthen your pelvic floor muscles, which can result in bigger, stronger, faster orgasms and can also improve urinary incontinence. In order to build those muscles it takes work—which means wearing the balls consistently over a number of weeks or months.

Most users are disappointed with Kegel balls because they expect them to be a sex toy that gives instant gratification. These folks weren't ready to dedicate themselves to a vaginal workout routine whose results take considerable time to manifest.

If you are one of the small percentage of women who does get turned on wearing the vaginal balls or you are dedicated to wearing them regularly to strengthen your orgasms down the road, they really are wonderful products.

There are so many options out there for bondage play. How do you know what's safe and high quality and what has the potential to break or be unsafe?

Any product can be unsafe depending on what you do with it. The level of quality one needs in a bondage device varies. For example, I may use a basic set of wrist cuffs to tie a partner's hands together, which is a perfectly acceptable use of the product. I should never, however, expect those same cuffs to support suspending my partner off the ground. It's important to not expect a product to handle more than it was designed for. Products that are safe for beginners may be dangerous for advanced play and vice versa.

I advise people who are exploring bondage (or any kind of kink) to fully educate themselves before playing. This is especially important if you intend to practice intermediate or advanced-level bondage.

Ropes tied improperly can cause nerve damage or asphyxiation, being restrained in certain positions can promote fainting or nausea, and a simple stumble in high heels can lead to severe injury if the sub can't catch herself because her hands are tied.

Taking classes, joining clubs and online communities or reading a few books can help kinksters develop the knowledge base they need to determine which products are safe for certain practices.

Are there any kinky toys that are just out-and-out unsafe, or does it all come down to proper usage and care?

Most of the time it does come down to proper usage and care. Again, it's really important not to expect a product to do or handle more than it was designed for. For products designed for kink and sex play, you can usually find product specifications and limitations in the instructions.

Risk assessment can be a bit more difficult to determine with pervertables. Since we aren't using these products for their intended purposes, we can't expect there to be a warning on the box. Also, with the recent interest in BDSM, there's a lot of bad information floating around causing people to think certain products are safe that really aren't. Zip ties and stockings are a prime example of this. Both products, when used for bondage, often keep tightening and don't loosen up. They can become so tight that it's near impossible to wiggle a safety scissor underneath to cut them off.

If you are intending to use a sex product or pervertable, head to a BDSM social site like fetlife.com first to ask other experienced kinksters to weigh in. Often there are helpful "beginning basics" safety guidelines on sites like this as well. Kink 101 classes are another great resource for learning about risks, safety procedures and what to do in an emergency.

What question has no one ever asked you on this topic, but you wish someone would?

Do BDSM scenes always have to be so serious and harsh? What if I don't like pain?

What would be the answer to that question?

Absolutely not! Kink does not have to be about being bad, receiving punishment and receiving pain. That's just one of many different scenarios. A BDSM scene can be tender and loving, it can include joking and laughter—it's whatever you make it. Just because we read about it in books or see stern behavior and pain in the movies, doesn't mean that's the only way.

Kink is a state of mind. From the dominant's point of view it's the act of taking someone on a mental journey by creating a mood and a scenario and adding physical elements that complement that journey. The details are what you and your partner make them. The sky really is the limit.

ANTHROPOLOGY

Donna George Storey

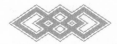

I was drawn to Andy from the moment I met him. No doubt part of it was his sky-blue eyes, his mischievous smile, and his large hands that looked like they could finger pussy for hours. But I think the real attraction was his profession. Andy was an anthropologist with a specialty in Indonesia. I'd been to London and Paris, but I've always nursed a yearning to explore someplace really exotic, even a little dangerous.

A month after we started dating, Andy asked if I wanted to go to a potluck party given by a fellow grad student in his department. It would be a chance to meet his friends—an interesting bunch, he promised—plus the food was guaranteed to provide a sensual education. Anthropologists always brought fascinating dishes they'd picked up from their world travels.

I said yes right away because I loved being with Andy, and I was tired of my usual English department get-togethers: pub-crawls and ironic Jane Austen teas.

The first five minutes of the party, however, were nothing to write home about. Andy and I handed over his homemade *nasi goreng* to our hostess, Natasha, who cordially informed me I could leave my coat in her bedroom while she got me some wine.

At that moment a new guest sauntered in, a leggy redhead named Penelope, who brought a dish of cilantro-and-cabbage dumplings she'd learned to cook in Shanghai. Perhaps it was because I was the exotic newcomer, but Penelope took an immediate liking to me. We went off to the bedroom together, chatting as if we were old pals.

I was about to toss my coat on the bed with the others, but Penelope's Chinese silk jacket wrinkled easily, and she suggested I hang mine up as well. As she reached for the door of the freestanding closet by the bed, I marveled at her anthropologist's boldness. Opening a stranger's closet without permission was definitely courting danger. Who knew what secrets lurked within?

But even I never expected the vision that greeted us as the door swung open.

"Wow," Penelope breathed.

My jaw dropped.

For Natasha's cabinet was indeed bursting with secrets. Or perhaps the better word would be "implements." Two black-leather paddles. A bouquet of riding crops. A square wooden board with a handle that looked like a pizza peel. An enema bag. Fur handcuffs. An assortment of leather straps, masks and studded collars.

"Oh, you've found my toy closet," our hostess said from the doorway.

I jumped guiltily.

In contrast, Natasha's smile was so innocent, we might have stumbled on her childhood collection of Barbies.

Then I noticed Andy standing behind her, his leather jacket draped over his arm. He, too, smiled benignly at the array of sexual playthings. Cultural relativism—surely the best defense in any awkward social situation.

I'd apparently mistaken Penelope's response for my own dismay, because she immediately launched into a nostalgic tale about the sexual predilections of a former boyfriend. He liked to give her enemas and was especially intrigued by how her abdomen got all swollen from the fluid. He'd rub his hands all over her belly, pressing lightly to make her squirm. Afterward, he always wanted anal sex.

Natasha nodded. "The two often go together."

"I've never been spanked, though," Penelope added.

"Would you like to be?" Natasha asked.

Penelope thought for a moment. "Why not?"

Natasha smiled. "That can be arranged."

My own belly contracted in sympathy, fear mixed with a decidedly sexual tingle of the taboo. I was half expecting the spanking to occur on the spot, which presented a dilemma. Should I stay and watch or run screaming back to Jane Austen?

Instead, Natasha and Penelope began to discuss their statistics class, while Andy pulled me away to meet a friend. I'd almost convinced myself the whole thing was a dream until half an hour later, when I spied Natasha leading Penelope back into the bedroom. She closed the door behind them.

Andy and I were seated on a nearby sofa, swapping travel tales with a fellow Southeast Asia hand, but my attention was focused solely on the hushed but tantalizing sounds floating through the door. I heard Penelope's voice rising in a question—I caught the words "bed" and "panties"—followed by a long stretch of silence. Had the spanking begun?

I nodded politely as the man droned on, but my eyes instinctively shifted back toward the bedroom. Then I did hear a *thwack*, then another and another. I cocked my ear for a cry or maybe pleading to stop—or go on—but I only heard a soft murmuring, then another few *thwacks*. A few minutes later, the door opened.

Penelope emerged, looking slightly flushed, but no worse for wear. "It feels like my butt just ate Indian food," she announced.

A few of the guests laughed, but the rest didn't even bat an eye. Apparently anthropologists were not easily shocked.

"Any other takers while I have the paddle out?" Natasha called from the doorway.

Andy arched an eyebrow at me. I gave him a no-fucking-way-in-hell frown.

But later, loose on wine, I got up the nerve to give Natasha what I thought was a provocative good-bye. "Thanks for the sex party."

"Oh, that wasn't a sex party," she purred. "If you're interested in a sex party, come back next Saturday."

Later, in the car, Andy said my eyes had popped open so wide, he was sure she'd smacked *me* on the ass.

In fact, my bottom was still smarting. English lit types might lead pedestrian lives, but we have good imaginations. "That was certainly an education for me, but you seemed to take it all in stride."

Andy shrugged. "Oh, I knew Natasha worked as a dominatrix on the side. We all do what we can to supplement our measly stipends."

"Have you ever been to one of her sex parties?"

"No. Would you like to go?"

My stomach fluttered with the same confused feeling—fear and desire all tangled together like a couple making love. I'd never been to Thailand or Borneo like Andy. The wildest thing I'd done in my timid little life was give him a blow job in the shower last week while I rubbed his tush crack with a soapy finger.

"If you really wanted to, I suppose I could go along and watch." I was aiming for cool, but my voice came out small and scared.

Andy glanced over at me. "I'll be honest with you, Julia. One of my old girlfriends was into mild BDSM. She couldn't come unless she was on top and I was spanking her ass and calling her a naughty slut. I enjoyed it, but that's because I liked to make her happy. My deepest desire now is to do whatever it is that makes *you* happy."

I sighed. "It all just seems so foreign to me."

"I know what you mean. The first few weeks I was teaching English in Jakarta, I was scared to death. But I'm glad I stayed. Traveling to a new place always stretches you, physically, mentally...and sensually."

The twinkle in his eyes definitely made me wonder where he might take me from here.

But Andy didn't mention the spanking party again. I was the one who couldn't get it out of my mind, especially when we made love. Entwined in his arms, I imagined I was back at Natasha's apartment, shamelessly opening the door to watch her spank Penelope's ass. Afterward, she smeared the now-blushing buttocks with chutney in languid, circular motions—a twist of fancy that was both absurd and strangely arousing. I saw myself taking her place, my body draped over the bed so Andy could snake an enema hose into my anus. I pictured him holding his inflamed tool to my cleansed opening, licking his lips in anticipation. But instead of fucking my virgin hole, he began to spank me across the ass with his boner, now brick red and massive like a knight's long sword. *Whack, whack.* I cried out with each blow and then gradually the sobs turned to pleas. *More, yes, more.*

Even out of bed, I found myself making excuses to brush my buttocks against Andy's crotch or bend over in front of him so he'd couldn't help but gaze at my ass. I purposely acted sassy so he'd call me a naughty girl. But I just couldn't get up the courage to ask him to spank me.

Then one day I happened to find myself at the local costume

shop. The selection of slutty outfits for women was impressive, but I immediately reached for the schoolgirl costume. Maybe actions would speak louder than words?

I handed him the bag with no explanation, a blush creeping over my cheeks.

"Is this a present for me?"

I nodded.

He pulled out the package, adorned with a smirking female dressed up in a plaid skirt and white blouse. His eyebrows shot up. "Thank you, but I'm afraid it's not my size."

I tried to laugh, but all that came out was a nervous cackle.

Andy studied my face. It took but a moment for the light to switch on in his eyes, but then again his job was the study of humankind. Grinning, he leaned close and whispered in my ear. "I can tell you're turned on by this, Julia. I can smell your wet pussy. Are you a naughty schoolgirl who gets hot and bothered by the idea of getting a good spanking?"

I inhaled sharply.

"I thought so. We'll need a safeword, so I'll know if I should stop. What should it be?"

"Anthropology." I'm not sure why that word popped into my head, but it seemed right.

He chuckled. "So it is. Now tell me what you did at school that deserves punishment."

He probably expected I'd have to make something up, but actually I did have one naughty secret in my own closet, a transgression from my undergraduate days when I worked at the campus library. Bored out of my mind, I'd sneak off to the quietest corner of C-Floor, shove my hand down my pants and bring myself to a muffled orgasm while the shelves of books looked on.

I'd never been caught, and I'd never told anyone. Until now.

"I...I hid in a quiet corner of the library, and I...I played with myself," I stuttered, my face flushing scarlet.

Andy clicked his tongue. "This calls for some serious intervention, Julia. Go change into your school uniform in the bedroom. Take off your panties, too. Because of course, you weren't wearing any when the librarian caught you masturbating in the stacks and sent you the principal's office for a good talking-to."

At first I doubted I could even stand up, my pulse was pounding so hard. But the sudden gush of desire drenching my panties brought me to my feet. Naughty as I felt, I didn't want to leave a wet spot on his sofa. I shuffled back to the bedroom, trembling like an addict desperate for her fix. I was still shaking as I tried on the middy blouse. The plunging neckline didn't even cover my bra, so I stripped everything off, wincing as the cheap cotton chafed my stiff, sensitive nipples. The plaid miniskirt fastened around my waist easily, but it was so skimpy, it barely covered my ass. The white thigh-highs only seemed to accentuate the problem.

Looking more like a stripper than a schoolgirl, I walked slowly back to the living room. I hoped the next part of the trip would be easier with an experienced traveler at my side.

Andy had moved over to his desk. His eyes glittered as he took in my short skirt and exposed cleavage. "Hello, Julia. Mrs. Beckwith informed me there was an incident in the library this afternoon." Though he was still in jeans and a T-shirt, his voice was all dressed up in a stuffy suit and tie.

I bowed my head. "Yes, Sir."

"In fact, I'm told you were found back among the English literature classics with your hand between your legs doing something unspeakable. Is that true?"

My first impulse was to deny it. Which was ridiculous, because I wanted what was coming. The sooner, the better.

"Yes, Sir," I whispered.

Andy's lips tightened with disapproval. "Perhaps you can tell me why you were so horny, you couldn't wait until you got home to do your dirty business?"

"I...I was thinking about my boyfriend, Sir."

"I see. Do you let him touch you between your legs?"

My cheeks felt scorched, and another flood of wetness coated my naked thighs.

"Well?"

"Yes."

"Well, this is a *very* serious matter, Julia. The disciplinary policy of the Academy no longer includes corporal punishment, but I must make an exception in this case. When the flesh errs, the body itself must be reprimanded. Come here and bend over."

I walked to him and placed my palms on the edge of his desk. As I leaned over, I noticed the unmistakable lump in his jeans. I pressed my lips together to hold back a smile.

Andy tucked the hem of my skirt up in the waistband, baring my asscheeks to the air. "Are you ready to suffer the consequences of your misdeeds, Julia?"

I whimpered assent.

With no further warning, Andy's palm met my buttocks with a satisfying crack. The stinging afterglow spread from my ass through my cunt and belly like a warm wave. He smacked me again. I cried out.

I hadn't invoked the A-word yet, but to my dismay, he stopped.

I waited, my ass burning, wondering if he was going to make me beg for more.

He cleared his throat. "How thoughtless of me to neglect the most important part. According to school policy, in order to truly learn her lesson, the student must be engaged in the offensive behavior while she is being punished. Therefore, I want you to diddle your clit while I continue to discipline you, Julia. Do you understand?"

"Yes, Sir." My voice cracked, but I obediently dipped my hand between my legs. My clit was so hard and big, I could have sworn it was dangling down between my legs like a small, satiny-pink cock. Andy waited until I got a good strumming going before he spanked me again. I gasped. The dueling sensations, shooting simultaneously from my clit and ass, made me forget everything else in the whole wide world.

Andy slapped me harder, once, twice, three times. He began to aim the blows directly on my asshole. I wiggled my ass like a puppy and begged, "Please, no," but I was nowhere near invoking the name of his exalted profession. In fact, I was in heaven.

"What are you thinking of now, Julia?"

"My boyfriend fucking my wet, swollen cunt," I choked out, my finger jiggling faster between my slick folds.

"Do you want to get fucked right now?"

"Yes, Sir, but..." I faltered, my throat tight with shame.

"But what?"

"Could you fuck my asshole instead?"

Andy clicked his tongue again. "You do have a dirty mind for such a prissy-looking miss. Did your boyfriend ever take you back there?"

"No, Sir, never."

"Too bad. If you were a naughty slut who got her ass fucked every day, I'd do it right now. But the first time requires special preparation. If you're a very good student this time, for our next session I'll bring an enema kit and some lube so I can punish your spanked, pink asshole properly."

I moaned again, but it wasn't from disappointment. His filthy words and the "confessions" he'd forced from my lips were sweet enough chastisement for now.

"Then fuck my wet pussy, Sir. Please." I opened my legs wider and tilted my ass up.

Laughing softly, Andy probed my vagina with the head of his cock, then buried himself in all the way to the root. He plowed me slowly, in and out, all the while maintaining a steady rain of blows on my buttocks. In this position, I felt every inch of him, his girth stretching my hole tight, the knob of his dick tickling my cervix. I was so sopping wet, his cock made sloppy, slurping sounds with each thrust.

"Tell me what a bad girl you are, Julia. Tell me how much you need to be punished."

"I'm bad. I play with myself in public. I bring dishonor to the Academy."

"That's right. You are a bad, bad girl. And now you must learn your lesson. Come on my cock, Julia. Milk your principal's prick with your horny, schoolgirl twat," Andy panted.

Then he reached around and pinched my nipples through the flimsy blouse. It was the last straw. My cunt spasmed around him and I screamed, "Fuck me, fuck me, oh yes!" Andy kept slapping my ass, the blows weakening as he grunted and shot his spunk into me.

For the longest time we stayed that way, floating together, cock in cunt, sweat and laughter, sweetness and spice all mixed together like a foreign elixir.

Later, when we'd wiped up and were sitting hand in hand on the sofa, I told Andy I thought I might be able to handle going to one of Natasha's sex parties after all.

"Really?" Eyes twinkling, he pulled me down over his lap and smoothed his big, warm hand over my bare buttocks. "I'm sure the other guests would agree your ass looks pretty in pink. But I have to warn you; fieldwork involves more than just showing up and watching. A serious anthropologist has to spend a lot of time preparing and practicing."

"I'll try to be a good student," I promised, pressing my mons against his thigh. Soon Andy and I would be off on another journey to some new and distant land that was really not so far away at all.

I had a feeling I was going to like it there.

CHAPTER FIVE

CULTURE AND ETIQUETTE

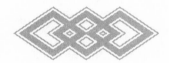

The first time I was invited to a kinky play party, I didn't actually realize what kind of event I'd said yes to. I thought it was a Western dress-up-style birthday party for a coworker of mine. While that probably sounds woefully naive, let me just say that, in my defense, the invitation did show a picture of a cowgirl with a whip saying, *Come celebrate twenty-five years of riding 'em hard and puttin' 'em away wet!* (Now that I've written that, I'm not sure if it helps or hinders my case....)

Either way, I dressed in my "best" Western outfit—as a girl who'd grown up riding horses, I had a lot of authentic gear, right down to the cowboy boots and my show hat, a pink leather number that I hadn't worn since I was about sixteen. I showed up, tipped my hat at the leather-clad woman who opened the door, and then had one of the more eye-opening experiences of my life. This mostly involved me standing in the kitchen with one or two other wide-eyed people in cowboy hats while everyone else get hot and heavy in the other rooms. It wasn't that I was uncomfortable with the amount of sex that was happening; it was that I wasn't prepared. I've never been that great at parties anyway, and this was an event for which I had no guidelines on how to act. Was I supposed to wait for someone to invite me to make out with him? Was it bad manners to just stand in the kitchen and look at the host's refrigerator magnets? While a few people said nice things about my spurs, it wasn't until much later that I realized the subcontext of their compliments. Even the photos that were shot of me that night show a girl with blonde braids and a huge hat, looking utterly confused and out of place while sitting on a strange man's semi-naked lap.

I wish someone had taken me by the hand that night and said, "Look, it's okay. If you want to make out with someone, that's cool. If you don't, it's also okay to stand here in the kitchen and eat all the chips instead."

Over the years, I've found that there are a whole lot of ways to play well with others. Sex-themed events come in all shapes and sizes. A party could be something as simple as a threesome or two couples swapping partners (neither of which are actually simple, of course, but they involve fewer people than a full-on dungeon party and so might be considered smaller and more private). Or it could be a large gathering held at a private home, large warehouse or private club, featuring hundreds of people, myriad play spaces and dozens of different sexual experiences all happening at the same time.

There are also sex-themed events that don't include any sex at all. Munches are a good example. These are informal social gatherings of people with an interest in BDSM, typically held in a restaurant or other public place. People attend with the goal of meeting like-minded kinksters to talk about anything of interest. Educational events are also great opportunities to spend time with other people who are interested in BDSM without engaging in sexual activities. Depending on where you live, you may find classes in rope bondage, anal sex, spanking and more. For those in rural or conservative areas, the Internet has opened up great opportunities for taking classes online.

Whether your public interest is in voyeurism, exhibitionism, play parties, dungeons, classes or something else, it's good to have some simple etiquette guidelines to help guide you. Here is what I wish I'd known during that first play party I went to, way back when:

1. Be Open-Minded

First and foremost, remember that this is a sexually themed event. You may see nude people, explicit sex, beatings, whippings, public humiliation, foot worship and an incredible number of other kinky activities. Whatever you see, whatever you hear, do your best not to react with shock, disgust, obvious surprise, or any other overt or negative emotion. If something freaks you out, politely excuse yourself and find something that seems like a better fit for you.

Note: This is not true if you see something happening that is clearly outside the bounds of consensual activity. In that case, the right thing to do is find someone in a position of power and tell him or her what you experienced.

2. No Touching (without permission)

It's considered very bad manners to touch people, toys, apparel, collars, play spaces, equipment or anything else at a public event without asking first.

This also extends to not touching yourself—if you're watching a scene without participating, be respectful. They're not there for your benefit or your pleasure. (As with all things, this is sometimes not true; if you've made an agreement ahead of time with the participants that you getting off is part of the scene or event, that's a different thing altogether.)

3. Be Polite
This seems obvious, but people who are nervous can sometimes do or say stupid things. If that's you, apologize. If that's someone else, give them the benefit of the doubt and a gentle reminder that manners count. If that doesn't fix the problem, it's time to find someone who will steer them in the right direction (usually out the door).

4. Be Honest
Nothing ruins an event faster than someone who's not being honest or who's purposefully hiding things. Don't hide your marital status, health, risk factors or anything else. Perhaps most important: don't be dishonest about your experience level. Those who play with you will take you at your word, and if you've never actually been whipped in public, there is no way that's going to end well for anyone involved.

5. Don't Puppy Dog
While puppy play is a positive element of many a sex party, puppy dogging—following someone around the event for a period of time— is likely to creep him out and send up red flags. If you're nervous or alone, don't glom onto someone hoping that person will take you under his or her wing. Your best option is to be honest and say that you don't know anyone yet. That way, people will want to introduce you and help you feel welcome. People in the community are incredibly welcoming to newcomers, especially those who are up-front about the fact that they're inexperienced.

6. Respect Privacy
Asking personal questions about where someone lives or works, what

her real name is, or what his email is are best held off until you establish a relationship with that person. Don't stalk other participants on Facebook or other social media sites after the event is over, and don't talk about the event with people who were not there. And don't take photos during the event unless explicitly invited by someone in charge; this is a serious breach of privacy that is not typically tolerated.

The reverse is also true—don't give out personal information to anyone that you don't already know and trust.

Get Your Passport Stamped: Go Public

1. Attend a Munch
If you've never attended a sex party, are generally shy, or just want to make some like-minded friends, try a munch. Almost all munches are advertised on the Internet; just search "munch" and your city, and you're likely to find anything that's available. (Again, if you live in a rural or conservative area, public events might be hard to find. Try a semiprivate site like fetlife.com, where people are more likely to post under the protection of the community.) Be yourself, be honest and open and see where it takes you.

2. Have a Virtual Event
If you're excited by the prospect of public play or of opening up your relationship, try a virtual event. This could be as simple as you and your partner watching a hot flick together and imaging that the third or fourth person is actually there with you. Describe what they're doing to you and your partner, how you're interacting with each other and what the experience is like. This kind of trial run can prepare you and your partner for the real thing, by bringing up any hidden issues and by getting some of your fear and worries out of the way.

The next step might be to meet someone via Skype or Google+ for a virtual play session. The distance created by the virtual medium can make everyone feel safer and more comfortable, while still providing that exciting sense of opening your relationship up to the public.

3. Go, But Don't Go Alone

When you're ready for your first public event, it's a good idea to go with a friend, partner or other trusted companion. Or ask a kinky couple that you know if they'd be willing to be your escort for the evening. This provides you with a sense of protection, takes the pressure off of you and ensures that you know at least someone at the event. Ideally, your friends will introduce you to their friends and acquaintances, and by the time the event is over, you'll be on your way to creating a kinky community of your very own.

GETTING OUT THERE:

Lee Harrington on Playing Well with Others

Lee Harrington is an internationally known sexuality/spirituality educator and award-winning author.

In your book, *Playing Well With Others*, you have a great chapter titled "Unicorns, Trolls and Other Creatures: Behavior Awareness in Kink Communities." What's the biggest mistake you see people making on their first forays into a kinky community?

People should be thinking twice about their approaches to social media. Face pictures may help make friends, but due to archiving, they might never truly be taken down. What they say in a chat room linked to them might come back years later. Their fetish list might "out" more about themselves than they want to share. Really consider what you put up online...the Internet has a long memory.

How do you begin to talk to your partner about exploring outside your relationship? Is there any right or wrong way to broach the topic?

Before even talking about being in an open relationship, make sure your own connection is solid. Swinging, polyamory and consensual nonmonogamy are not the best ways to repair or "fix" a shaky dynamic.

Contracts seem to be a pretty hot topic among the newly kinky right now, perhaps due to their appearance in recent erotic novels. Are contracts a necessary part of negotiating or are they just one of many tools in a kinky person's toolbox?

Contracts are just one option for how to communicate what all parties are interested in and how they will get those desires met. But there are so many more ways to share your desires and make sure everyone is on the same page—and a lot of the other ideas can be sexier! Curling up in bed and whispering sweet nothings, filling out questionnaires of kinky ideas and sharing them with each other, having a nice conversation over dinner, trying one thing out and debriefing afterward before trying anything else out... I encourage folks to find the format that will help them feel safe, heard *and* connected.

Do you have any advice for the kinky introvert when it comes to jumping into the kink community?

Just because you are introverted or shy does not mean you can't have fun in the kink community. Consider getting a funny T-shirt or sexy outfit to encourage folks to come to you, instead of having to approach others right away. Try making friends online before going to events, or write a little note to an event host asking for introductions to folks when you get there. And...take time for yourself. It is completely fine to show up to a party and watch. You don't have to dive into the deep end on your first night out.

How has the Internet changed the ability to connect with the kink community, for both good and bad?

The Internet has brought so many folks out to dip their toes into not just their bedroom passions, but the broader communities as well. Classes and events are more accessible, and social gatherings/munches can be looked up with a few search engine words (or a profile on a kinky social media site). Online anonymity, however, means that you don't have the same interpersonal connections that help vet people who are coming in, and who you are learning from. The intimacy of small parties is being replaced with massive conferences. But the access also provides safety for getting information—quite the mixed bag. I'm grateful for the new information myself…resources can be found almost anywhere in the world.

What question has no one ever asked you on this topic, but you wish someone would?

Am I expected to have sex with people that I do other forms of kinky play with?

What would be the answer to that question?

You get to make choices for yourself about who you play with, and what the word *play* means to you. Some folks like adding bondage to the existing sexual interactions they've already had. Some people like going to a party and getting spanked, but don't want to have any sort of genital contact with their pickup partner. Others love giving floggings one night with their spouse, but have sex be something for a non-kinky night. There are people who may never have sex with their kinky play partners. Before you play, make sure all parties know what "play" means to them, and whether sex, or sexual contact, is part of their "play" definition.

PETTING ZOO

Rachel Kramer Bussel

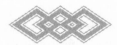

When you truly love someone, you'll do anything for him and vice versa. That goes a long way toward explaining what I was doing dressed in five-inch, shiny leather boots, my voluptuous body poured into a corset, wearing a long black wig and holding a chain, which was attached to a collar, which was attached to my husband, Mason. The collar was all he had on, by my command. But my command was, ultimately, a response to his request, one of many such pleas, during our increasingly heated role-playing sessions. There he was, his thirty-two-year-old, hairy, oversized body on full display not just to me but also to a whole roomful of kinky people, mostly women. I smiled as I stared down at my pet for the night. I'd gotten used to the role I now proudly played, but getting there took some time, and a whole lot of love.

We'd been married for just over a year before somehow, my buff, seemingly butch hubby, who loved to race his motorcycle when we ventured out of the city, who was proud of his home-cooked steaks, who grew a beard and disdained the "pretty boys" who got proper haircuts rather than having their wives trim their tresses, revealed to me one day that what he wanted most was to worship at my feet; to be my servant, my slave, my pet. Inside his macho exterior lurked the heart of a pure submissive. He'd never done it, but he'd apparently spent the last six months thinking about submitting, about giving it up to me, his wife who usually could be found on all fours taking his gigantic cock in her pussy and once in a while in her ass. Instead of my bending over, he wanted me to tower over him. Okay, there was a little more that he wanted, like the chance to lick anonymous women's pussies, to be used like a toy, but all that only worked if I was the one "making" him do it.

It was a revelation, the first time he said it. My mind whirred with this new side of him, more surprised that he'd kept the fantasy from me than that he possessed it in the first place. It's not like we were shy and retiring, or never talked about sex; we made sure to keep our sex life as lively as it had started out, after our whirlwind, very hot romance, which included joining the mile-high club, plenty of phone sex and all sorts of sharing of dirty talk. I'd thought that in the year and a half we'd been together we'd unearthed each other's every secret. Not that I was bored or anything, but I felt like we'd grown into ourselves, our marriage, and were at a point where we could finish each other's sentences. But apparently, there were things I still had to learn. I was in the middle of spinning a tale of me punishing an imaginary wisp of a girl I'd bring home, telling her how she'd sucked his cock the wrong way, when something shifted.

"You're gonna punish her really hard, right? Spank her ass?" His voice betrayed his excitement. The truth is, we weren't really entertaining the idea of a threesome, but it was the fantasy, the image, the idea that we were both responding to. I wasn't opposed to adding another woman, or man, into the mix someday, but not just yet. First I wanted to see how far we could take our own filthy fantasies.

"Yeah, you want to see that, right?" As I was talking, he turned over, and there was his ass, right before me. I cupped his cheeks and before I knew it I was giving Mason a demonstration of just what I would do to our mystery girl.

"You want me to tie you up and have women come over and sit on your face, is that what you're telling me?" I asked him one night as I myself straddled his pretty face, giving him his fill of his favorite meal. By then, I'd gotten used to our favorite fantasy scenario, had started to think of myself the way Mason thought of me, at home and when I was outside of it. I'd never been with anyone, man or woman, who was so eager for oral, even me, and I can't get enough cock down my throat when I'm with the right person. His enthusiasm in turn engendered my own, but what I loved most was feeling him tremble when I talked dirty to him, when I spun tales of all the wicked things I was discovering I'd like to do to him.

I'm not naturally the dominant type; I haven't always taken the pride I do now in seeing a man cowering before me, but Mason has turned me into the kind of woman who loves a cruel smile, a harsh look, who loves to fling her boot out and watch him scurry to pull it off. That attitude has carried over into my professional life, where I've risen up the ranks of the cosmetics company I started at as a secretary; now I'm a vice president.

I thought for a moment about my climb up the corporate ladder as I watched Mason crawl on the ground, surrounded by beautiful women. This was his dream come true, and watching his ass, his middle-aged, hairy ass, the one I thought of as mine to enjoy, made me smile. In a way, I was doing this for him, but in so many other ways, I was doing it for me. I stood taller when he got on his knees. I got wet when he groveled, and I got a thrill out of seeing the other women coo over him. He truly was like a pet, or a toy, and thinking of him that way only made me love him more. I also knew he'd never be the type to cheat; why would he, when I allowed him to lick all the pussies he wanted? Well, that's not entirely true.

When he crawled over to me and I leaned down so he could kiss his way up from my cleavage to my neck, and then he whispered, "Mistress?" in my ear, I had a feeling I knew what was coming.

"Yes, pet?"

"There is a woman who I'd like to play with. She's over there and she has a beautiful flogger and…"

"And what?" I prompted, knowing it would be a struggle for him to praise her without somehow denigrating me. Watching his mouth open and close amused me, and aroused me. I was pleased to find that I wasn't just doing this for him, because that one-sided type of sacrifice can ruin any relationship, even a kinky one.

"And…she's looking for someone to torture."

"And you think you'd be just the right someone?" I asked him.

"Because I…" he paused. "Because I want to try something new. You know I'm devoted to you, Mistress, one hundred percent. I want everyone to watch and see how much I can take, and be jealous of you that you get to take home such an obedient boy." I smiled. It was a good answer, a way of spinning his own urgent desire into something that would give me some street cred, too. I wanted Mason to be happy, because without that, what was the point of our marriage? And by now I was curious to see what exactly would happen when I let him roam and play.

"Okay, you have my permission, but you better be done in half an hour, or I'm going to drag you out of here by your hair and make you crawl around outside on the street wearing only what you're wearing now." Of course I'd never do such a thing, but it was plausible enough that he didn't need to know my true intentions. I could tell that my "threats" were part of what got him excited, and doing that for him in turn made me feel like a good wife, not in a traditional way, but in my way. Yes, call me crazy, but I saw my act of issuing bold threats of bodily harm as almost, well, romantic.

Mason was overjoyed, and if he'd had a tail, it would've been wagging. Instead, his cock bobbed up and down. "But you know that your cock belongs to me, right? We don't have to get you a cage for it, do we?" I reached down and stroked his balding head, my gentle hand playing good cop to my words' bad cop.

"Of course not. I'd never let another woman touch me there." Mason sounded almost offended that I'd even mention it.

"Okay then, you head on over, I'll be by to watch soon. Be good for her; I don't want to hear any complaints." I unclipped the chain but kept the collar on him, smiling as I watched him go, then stood and surveyed my surroundings. I'd slowly turned into the kind of woman who belonged in such a setting, a woman who could walk proudly, even in five-inch heels, and not feel self-conscious about her breasts practically hanging out of a corset. It's taken me a while to become comfortable with my voluptuous body, to not want to whittle it down to a size six or four, but to be proud of its ten or twelve. Even with Mason's love and devotion, it wasn't until we started coming to parties like these that I truly saw what the extra weight could do for me, how it helped me to tower over men like Mason, how it made the snap of a whip sound that much louder, how my heft made me more of a woman, not less.

I owed that to him, though I'd never quite gotten around to telling my husband that. He didn't need to know my every innermost thought; I'd learned that that was one of the keys to a happy marriage. I walked toward him and found him with a bright-red butt plug sticking out of his ass, one that looked on the large side. I knew he'd never worn one before; we'd talked about it, but that was as far as it had gotten. His lips were wrapped around the heel of a shiny black boot, which was attached to a strikingly beautiful woman with long, glossy black hair, shiny pink lips and layers of mascara. She looked like she was in her early twenties, and for a moment, jealousy threatened to undo my inner goddess.

But then I walked closer and saw the look of joy on Mason's face as he sucked, his eyes closed. I stepped back when a loud cracking sound issued right near me; it was a whip, landing on Mason's ass. He let out a yelp, but went right back to sucking the boot. The woman looked up at me and winked, the perfect action to pacify my nerves. She seemed to know that the man sucking on her boot was mine, all mine, and that she was only borrowing him. He was her pet not for the night, but for the moment.

"Is this your owner, slave?" she called down to him, pointing toward me.

Mason's face flushed red before he said, "Yes, Ma'am, that's Mistress Stephanie." He'd called me "Ma'am" and even "Mistress," but never "Mistress Stephanie," like a proper title.

"Is my property behaving?" I asked, just as the woman with sleek white hair sent another crack of the whip against his butt.

"Oh yes, he is," the first woman said, running the tip of her shoe along his cheek. He smiled up at her while I surveyed the scene. Just then I spied a young man who looked like he could use a spanking. I knew this because he was holding a somewhat forlorn sign saying SPANK ME. IT'S MY BIRTHDAY. If Mason could indulge, so could I. "I'll be back," I said, and knew Mason would be curious about where I'd gone. I didn't need to watch him at work to know how grateful he would be to me for granting him this excursion.

"What's your name and how old are you?" I kept my voice husky and severe.

"George. I'm twenty-one."

"A baby, are you? Well, George, that's my husband right over there," I said, pointing toward Mason. George gasped, then looked back at me. "Maybe someday you'll be lucky enough to be married to a woman like me, but right now, I have a little time on my hands and I wouldn't want to see a birthday boy like you not get the spanking you deserve. I'm going to give you one smack for each year you've been alive, and you're going to thank me for them, loudly. You're going to say, 'Thank you, Mistress Stephanie.' Do you understand me?"

"Yes, Mistress Stephanie," he said, and proceeded to position himself across my lap. I pulled down his pants and gave him a nice, firm slap. The sound echoed in the air and I soon became enamored of the way this lithe young man reacted to each smack. I didn't forget about Mason, exactly, but he wasn't foremost in my mind. I knew he was in good hands, or feet, as it were.

"Louder!" I roared as I reached the eighth blow, wanting to make sure Mason heard, wanting him to know that while I was here mostly at his behest, this wasn't all about him. Pets don't control their owners. By twelve, George's ass was very red, and very warm. My palm was stinging, so I took more time between slaps, using that time to tease his asshole with my index finger, to pinch his enflamed cheeks, to dig my nails into his back. Spanking him was giving me all sorts of ideas of what I wanted to do with Mason.

I pictured myself punishing Mason—it didn't matter for what— and that added extra vigor to my smacks. The last few were extra loud and extra hard, and when I let George stand up and kiss my hand, he was breathing heavily. I walked back over to check on Mason. He had a handprint across his cheek, and was sitting with his legs tucked beneath him, waiting for me.

"Did he behave?" I asked the Mistress whose name I hadn't caught.

"Well enough," she said.

"And?" I prompted Mason.

"Thank you very much," he said to each of the women he'd had the pleasure of bottoming to.

"Now it's time to go home. And you're going to wear just your rubber shorts." At his look, I smiled. "Yes, of course I brought them for you; I wouldn't let you walk around with your cock, the one that belongs to me, hanging out. You can also wear your shoes." I could tell he wanted to protest, that he thought maybe I was taking our D/s arrangement a little too far, but I'd granted him his wish, and he was going to grant me mine. That was how things worked in this brave new kinky world.

"Yes, Mistress Stephanie," he said. I grabbed his cock and led him toward our bags, squeezing just a little harder than I needed to. And I liked the way it felt. Our night was far from done, but we'd each gotten something that we'd wanted. I may not be naturally dominant, but I'm a fast learner. And I have the best teacher a Mistress could ask for.

CHAPTER SIX

HEALTH AND WELL-BEING

There's an old adage that your biggest sex organ is your brain. And while that may seem true for many of us—I know it certainly seems true for me most of the time—perhaps the real truth is that our biggest sex organ is our entire body. From the subtly of our synapse-firing brains and our incredibly sensitive noses to the in-your-face sexuality of our shakealicious booties, our bodies are built for sex.

When you start reading about BDSM and health, you'll notice a lot of articles about caring for yourself right before, during and after sex. Words like *aftercare* pop up a lot, as do conversations about emergency situations. These are all important elements of caring for your kinky self (and we cover some of them in the next section), but I would argue that taking care of yourself all of the time, in your everyday life outside of your sexual self is a vital and often overlooked element of BDSM health and safety.

Taking care of your body doesn't mean you have to run a marathon, be in perfect shape, go on a diet or anything drastic. In fact, sometimes taking care of yourself just means sitting still, getting in touch with your body and mind and figuring out what you need to be healthy and well. One of the great things about BDSM is that it fits everyone. You don't have to be a certain size, a certain shape or a certain anything to enjoy kinky sex. There's no willing body that's the wrong size for a pair of ankle cuffs, no shape of butt that can't be caressed or spanked, no length of penis that won't feel right at home in a gorgeous leather cock ring. Sure, we're all different and our bodies react differently to different sexual experiences, but that's something to embrace, not to run away from.

Me, I'm a klutz, first and foremost, so over the years, a fair number of my sexual interactions have started out something like this:

Me: "Ow! Crap!"

Partner: "But I didn't even touch you yet."

Me: "I just walked into the table on my way to bed."

Partner: "You know, if you were tied down, you wouldn't walk into things every five seconds."

Me: "I'll get the bondage tape!"

But your body isn't the only thing that can get banged up during kinky sex. Your mind is vulnerable too. How we feel about ourselves in relation to our sexual interests can affect our day-to-day experiences in and out of the bedroom. This is especially true of kinksters, where the pressure to be "normal" can be profound. Walk through the world with a kink or two in your bag of tricks, and you've probably also walked through the world with an equal helping of guilt, shame, distress or other negative emotions about your perversion.

Over the years, kink has gotten a bad rap—and not just from the places you might expect. Many religions, of course, have a lot of negative things to say about kink (and truly, about sex in general). Some of your family members, friends, partners and ex-partners might look down upon your interests—not to mention society as a whole.

The health profession hasn't always been as open-minded as it is today either. Doctors reported abuse, even if a patient tried to explain that she really liked having her ass caned hard enough to leave those welts and bruises. Many kinky activities, including fetishism and sadism, were once listed by the American Psychiatric Association as mental disorders. (That hasn't gone away entirely, however. The current *Diagnostic and Statistical Manual of Mental Disorders* lists "paraphilic disorders," such as sexual masochism disorder. However, to be diagnosed with one of these noncriminal sexual disorders, you must be experiencing personal distress or otherwise be unhappy about your particular kink.)

For so long, BDSM was so misunderstood that it was common practice, even among psychologists, to assume that anyone with kinky proclivities was mentally ill. The belief was that the desire to be spanked, tied up, dominated or otherwise have "non-vanilla" sex correlated strongly with childhood abuse, rape and mental disorders, and thus those experiencing or acting on these desires were more likely to be depressed or mentally unstable. Thankfully, this has turned out to not be true. In fact, a study published in the *Journal of Sexual Medicine* in 2013 found that BDSM practitioners are likely to have high levels of mental health. According to the study's findings, kinksters are often less neurotic, more open to new experiences, less sensitive to rejection and have a higher subjective sense of well-being.

This all makes sense, if you think about it. We know that having a sex life is good for our mental health. Having a great sex life that meets our specific needs—a kinky sex life for a kinky person—is likely to be even better for our emotional well-being.

Of course, that doesn't mean that there aren't some mental difficulties involved with coming to terms with our kinky sides. You might struggle with self-acceptance, societal, familial or religious pressures to conform, a sense of "otherness," or myriad other issues. If you've been attacked, raped or assaulted in any way, there's a chance that you're still carrying those emotional scars as well. None of these responses are bad or unusual; they are, in fact, all very normal responses to the difficulties that life throws at us. While our emotional vulnerabilities may or may not have anything to do with our interest in BDSM, it's a good idea to tackle them head-on outside of a kinky space. Being involved in BDSM experiences can bring up deep, unsettling emotions that can rock us to our core, no matter how mentally stable we are. Having a lifestyle that supports good mental health will allow you to better communicate your emotional needs and reactions, and can help you stay balanced during tough scenes. Thus, it's important to accept and recognize any emotional struggles that you're having, and to find your own best solutions—whether that's professional help, a supportive community, a caring partner or a mix of all of these—so that you can truly enjoy your sexual experiences with a minimum of psychological stress.

Taking care of your body and mind for the long haul is one of the most important gifts you can give yourself and your sex life. Focusing in on your physical and emotional needs right before, during and after sex play is an equally important gift.

Before starting anything, make sure that you've disclosed any pertinent information about your physical and emotional health. Kinky sex has the potential to put unique strains on the body and mind, and it's important that everyone involved has the medical information that they need to make good decisions. Do you have a heart condition, diabetes or high blood pressure? Are you allergic to latex, spermicides or another material that's commonly used during play? Do you take medications with possible implications for certain activities? Bad joints are another issue to watch for, especially during bondage, holding kneeling positions, or other activities that put strain on the places where our bodies bend. Do you have any emotional triggers that partners should avoid or look out for? Most of these aren't issues that should keep you from your desired form of play (unless, of course, your doctor says otherwise) but keeping everyone informed will decrease your risk of additional injury and help ensure that kinky sex is a fun, healthy experience for years to come.

Before you begin playing is also a good time to make an assessment of your own physical and emotional needs. Make sure you've eaten, taken any necessary medications, gone to the bathroom and taken care of anything else that needs to be done, so when the times comes to play, you can jump in without any worries.

During sex, communicate any issues right away. If you start to feel dizzy, short of breath, in "bad pain" (unwelcome, unexpected pain, as opposed to "good pain"—the kind of pain that brings feelings of pleasure), say something immediately and stop.

Aftercare is the period after a kinky sexual experience where you spend time with each other. I kind of think of it as returning to the "real world"—you're coming down from the endorphin high and assessing things. How do you feel, mentally and physically? How does your partner feel? What do each of you need now—food, water, release, sleep, ice packs, bandages, cuddle time, a mix of all of those things?

BDSM is a custom-fit experience, made just for you. You, your brain and your body become partners in a complex dance. If you listen, it will lead you in the direction that it needs to go for its best self. If you're reading this, then the chances are good that one of the directions your body often leads you is toward some type of BDSM sex—that, for kinky people, IS an important part of our physical and mental health.

Get Your Passport Stamped: Self Care

1. Look at Your Lifestyle

If kinky sex is a small but important part of your entire well-being, then it's probably not a bad idea to explore the other aspects of your general physical and mental health the same way you explored your kinks. What foods and drinks make you feel the best? What type and amount of physical activity leaves you feeling refreshed and inspired? What other types of play are important for your emotional joy? Do you get the amount of sleep that works for you? The tricky part about health is that there is no right answer—no one else can look at you and say, "You need to lose/gain five pounds, eat only vegetables and sleep ten hours a night in order to be your best kinky self." It's different for each of us and ever evolving.

2. Know Your Body

An attentive partner will pay attention and pick up on your physical and emotional responses during a particular scene, but no one knows you the way you do—and no one should be expected to. No matter how close you are to your partner, the onus is on you take good care of the body that you'll be putting through these strenuous experiences. Pay attention to your own body, both in and out of sex play. Be honest with yourself—the body you had at twenty that bounced back from anything isn't the body you have at forty. Old injuries, weaknesses and sore spots can all rear their heads without warning during a scene, so be prepared and talk to your partner(s) about it beforehand. Denial of your body's weaknesses is a quick way to additional injuries.

3. Protect Your Body

Your body is yours, and it doesn't belong to anyone else (unless you've willingly given it to them for their own personal pleasure, and hopefully yours too).

But on a more serious note, don't give your body to anyone that you don't want to. This seems obvious, I know, but I mean it in more than a physical sense. Saying no to sex or other physical contact is just one part of protecting and supporting your body. The other part is saying no to unwanted emotional contact. We live in a society where people feel comfortable commenting on other people's physical forms all the time. They catcall people on the street, tell strangers to smile, and comment on how hot or fat or slutty or doable someone is without thinking twice. While you can't make that go away, you can take whatever action feels best for you: turning a deaf ear, creating change, reporting perpetrators, saying no or finding another way to keep them from touching you, physically or emotionally.

4. Choose Good Practitioners

Carefully screen your doctors, mental health professionals, massage therapists and other care providers who will be in contact with your body and mind on a regular or semi-regular basis. Ideally, try to find practitioners who are kink- and sex-positive, who are knowledgeable about the topic and who can be an advocate for your kinky lifestyle. If you can't find supporters in the professional field (and even today they can be difficult to find, especially in conservative areas or small towns), aim for someone who isn't negative or reactionary about those bruises on your arm or the cut marks along the insides of your thighs. This is especially important for your OB-GYN or whichever doctor takes care of your sexual health. If you're struggling to find someone, ask people you know in the kinky community for suggestions or search online for kink-friendly doctors. Often, doctors or medical groups that are listed as GLBT-friendly are also kink-friendly (they just don't advertise as such).

The National Coalition for Sexual Freedom has a comprehensive directory of kink-aware professionals at ncsfreedom.org/resources/kink-aware-professionals-directory/kap-directory-homepage.html and the American Medical Association has a wonderful, free publication called "Beyond Whips and Chains" designed to introduce doctors to kinky patients. It can be a good icebreaker for you and your doctors, if you have concerns about their stance on BDSM: amsa.org/AMSA/Homepage/EducationCareerDevelopment/AMSAAcademy/SHLC/Additional.aspx

Whatever you do, if you need care, don't delay out of fear of repercussion or stigma. And be as honest as you can about your experiences. If an injury occurred during sex and you say it was from a football game, you're crippling your doctor's ability to provide you with the best care.

DOES A BODY GOOD:

Dr. Lynk on Staying Well

Dr. Lynk is a Doctor of Physical Therapy and Certified Strength and Conditioning Specialist.

In your experience in the health and fitness field, what's the biggest advice that you can give people who want to make a change in their lifestyle to improve their kinky experiences?

Do what you enjoy and know why you are doing it for you. Change, particularly changing your lifestyle, is difficult, time consuming, and has to be something you are doing for you. By engaging in activities that you enjoy, you are far more likely to do them and to keep doing them to make a sustainable change. Secondly, if you understand why you are doing something and what the change will mean for you on an emotional level, you will be more likely to succeed with your change. Too many times people (and I am just as guilty) attempt to change for reasons that are not their own or they do not understand why the change is important for them. As a result, they likely will not be able to make or sustain the change. The classic example is weight loss. Every year, millions of people get gym memberships to lose weight as a part of a New Year's resolution. The majority of those people will no longer be going to the gym in a month. Now, there are a multitude of reasons for this that may extend beyond motivation and enjoyment, but many stop going because they do not enjoy it or are lacking appropriate understanding of why they want to change. Once you understand the "why" and what you enjoy, all that is left to do is take action to change.

Let's talk about injury prevention: what can kinksters do to decrease their risk of getting injured during play?

Due to the wide variety of activities in which one can engage in the world of kink, injury prevention can be a little complex. However, one thing is very consistent in how the human body operates. The body does not like pain. Now, I know that is a very controversial statement given a large number of kink activities are based in pain, so allow me to explain. First, when I am referring to pain in this case I am referring to "bad pain" like knee pain, lower back pain, headaches, nerve pain, et cetera. When it comes to dealing with injuries, pain is the body attempting to tell you to stop whatever movement or position that is causing the pain. If we do not make a change or are unable to make a change to stop the pain, then the body will change how it moves and engages with the world in an attempt to lessen or entirely avoid the pain. Those changes to our movement are mostly unconscious and more or less always detrimental. With this concept in mind, the advice I would give to anyone regarding injury prevention or injury management would be to avoid or lessen pain as often as necessary to allow the body to heal and avoid chronic changes in movement patterns that may be harmful. If there is no way to avoid or change the pain, then you need to seek out the care of a professional to assist you.

If you already have an injury, what can you do to manage stress and pain, both before and during kinky sex?

For people who are in pain, the above concept still applies. If you engage in an activity that causes more pain, then you want to find a position or movement that helps to reduce pain. Once that movement or position is determined, then that can be utilized before, during and after any activity. If there is no way to change your pain, then you

SHANNA GERMAIN

should seek out the care of a knowledgeable professional to assist with managing and reducing your pain.

What specific health and fitness suggestions can you give for those who are into more strenuous BDSM activities, such as bondage, spanking or caning?

If you are operating on the more strenuous end of kink activities such as extreme bondage or heavy impact, then you have to be more mindful of bad pain. These ideas can also be applied to anyone else regardless of whether they are participating in strenuous activities. Prior to the scene, I would recommend being active to warm up the tissues of the body, which may allow them to sustain less injury.

Of more importance is learning how to breathe through your diaphragm. Taking a breath is typically the first thing we do when we are born and it is critical to be able to function at optimum capacity. If you are about to engage in an activity that is going to push the limits of your body, you want to be at your best in order to handle what is about to happen. Inside of more intense activity, being able to control your breathing allows for a focal point for the mind, but also provides a type of central anchor point for the body to stabilize from. Having an efficient breathing pattern is the easiest place to start with improving how your body functions and impacts your movement patterns, core stability and nervous system, to name a few.

In order of importance for the body to function, oxygen is first, second is water. Hydration is critical for the body to function, perform, sustain and heal itself. Without it, everything becomes less efficient and more dysfunctional. Third is sleep. Although we still do not understand fully why we need sleep, we do know that we need sleep more than we need food to survive. Getting good quality sleep positively impacts just about all aspects of health.

FICTION

GETTING IT RIGHT

Teresa Noelle Roberts

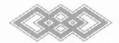

Heather knelt down at her boyfriend Jesse's feet. It wasn't something she normally did—at least not outside the bedroom or wherever they happened to get their kink on—but it was a safe position from which to say what she was about to say, a safe position in which to feel small and soft and submissive, nervous and wet at the same time.

Jesse hit the remote, obviously figuring news delivered by a kneeling lover would be more interesting than anything CNN had to offer. "Yes?"

She took a deep breath, took Jesse's hands, looked into his eyes. "I want to feel the cane again. Please."

He raised an eyebrow. "Are you sure?"

"Yes…" A split second's hesitation. "I hate being afraid. The longer we wait, the more I'll build it up as a big deal in my mind. So I figure we just do it—but do it right this time."

"That's my brave girl." He raised their joined hands to his lips and kissed hers, letting his tongue dart out to tease her knuckles. "I love you."

She grinned, a little weakly, trying to hide the way she was lurching between arousal and terror. "I love you too, but it's not unselfish, Jesse. I need the closure. That was a weird night, and I need to get past it. And besides," she added, hoping she sounded more confident than she felt, "I bet it'll be fun when we're not both being stupid."

He smiled. "Stupid's the word. We both know better than to play when we're mad."

"This time we'll do it right."

Almost a month ago, UPS had delivered the cane they'd ordered. They excitedly made plans for a lovingly kinky evening experimenting with the new toy, starting light and working up, since while Jesse had some prior experience wielding a cane, Heather knew only that it sounded hot in erotica.

There must have been something nasty in the air, though. On the night they'd planned for their cane experiment, Heather came home grouchy after a bad day at work to find Jesse just as irritable. They couldn't remember, afterward, how it had started, but they got into an argument after dinner, the kind that would never reach a resolution because it wasn't actually about anything.

The only points they agreed on was that Heather had started it—and they both wanted to stop it. For some reason, at one in the morning on a weeknight, it had seemed like a great idea to use that new cane for a punishment scene and work things out that way.

Maybe it wouldn't have been such a bad idea if they'd ever done a punishment scene before, or if Heather hadn't dropped so hard, worn by pain and emotion, that she forgot to use her safeword before Jesse broke skin. Under the circumstances, it had ended in tears, and not the good, cathartic kind, but the kind that left both of them wondering if they were both crazy to be playing games with pain and power.

A few nights of attempting to be vanilla had convinced them they'd be even crazier if they didn't play those games. But the cane stayed buried deep in the toy bag and neither of them had been sure it would come out again.

Until Heather asked.

This time they pulled out all the stops. This time the room was full of flickering vanilla- and cinnamon-scented candles, adding a medieval, almost religious air to Jesse's plain bedroom.

This time there was no anger, no exhaustion, no confusion, just lust and love and, at least on Heather's side, a lot of sexy anxiety. Under the angst and foolishness, that first time, she'd caught hints that she would like the cane under better circumstances.

But it still scared her.

And Jesse saw her fear and helped her through it.

They necked like teenagers on the couch before moving into the bedroom and kissing and caressing some more, so Heather was wet and quivering even before she began to undress.

This time, Jesse sat on the bed and put her over his knee, as he had their first night together. Starting with light, loving smacks that sent the blood rushing, stimulating her skin, stimulating her sex, he warmed her up until she was pushing her backside up to meet his hand. Then he stepped it up a little, cupping the sweet spot of her ass with each blow, half watching the color turning from creamy to pink to almost red, half watching Heather's reaction, the pleading little yelps, the squirming, the way she parted her legs, letting loose some of her aroused musk.

"How I can resist that invitation?" Jesse stroked her vulva, then slapped it lightly, teasingly. His fingers came away wet and slick. "Now that's what I like to see," he said, his voice breathy, smoky.

He pulled her up, kissed her, lingering and deep. "Now lie on your back," he commanded. "I have a vision."

Then he started arranging her.

He arched her over so her thighs rested on her chest and told her to hold herself in place with her arms.

He tucked several pillows under her, raising her ass. "Perfect," he said. "I have a gorgeous target, but I can watch your face."

He didn't add *in case you need to safeword and can't find your voice*, but he didn't need to.

"I can't hold this," Heather said. "I'm afraid I'll move at just the wrong time."

"That's what rope's for."

Slowly, sensually, he tied her that way, ass in the air, pussy open and exposed, muscles straining. Deliciously helpless, and the embrace of the ropes made her feel safer.

Juice poured from her pussy.

Jesse lay on the bed, buried his face in her wet, exposed slickness, and took a deep breath as if the scent intoxicated him. "Yum." He began to lick.

"Jesse...what are you doing?" Heather was genuinely confused. The last cane scene had been so rough his gentleness caught her off guard.

"Making you come," he said simply, before going back to what he'd been doing.

Already wet, her pussy flooded as he tongued her, and he licked as if trying to get every drop. Of course this just made her produce more. At first, though, he kept his attentions on the lips, keeping away from her clit.

She mewled, tried to squirm to get her clit under his questing tongue, but there was only so far she could move in her current position, especially with his weight on her. He licked and licked, pausing only to take his hard cock into his hand and say, "See what you're doing to me already? I love having power over you. I don't need to hurt you to have power over you, just offer you pleasure and the possibility of more. But I want to hurt you a little. Do you want that?"

"Yes, I do. But what you're doing right now...it's so good."

"Come for me," he whispered, just before he put his tongue where she craved it.

And she did.

While she was still riding the waves of orgasm, he slipped away, picked up their favorite leather slapper.

A few good whacks took her butt from pink to red—and pushed her over to another orgasm. "That's my girl," he said, pride in his voice. "That's the good naughty girl I love. Are you ready?"

When she nodded, he reached for the cane.

Heather took a deep breath, bracing herself for the onslaught of pain. She thought she could bear it now, after all the pleasure and tenderness, but when she heard the cane hiss through the air toward her, she held her breath, tensed her muscles in fear, waiting for the fire.

A tap. A very stingy tap, but a tap. It felt like nothing at first, then like a long paper cut, stinging, but not too intense.

Then fire coiled through her, merged into the heat between her legs and deep inside her body.

She'd figured that after two orgasms in quick sensation, she was somewhere in the sensation Himalayas.

No, she'd only been in the foothills. Erotic energy snaked through her, setting her alight, carrying her higher. "More," she groaned, straining against the ropes that held her safe, unable to articulate clearly the strange but beautiful sensations inside her.

The next blow was harder but sweeter, pushing her deeper. The next took her even farther. "Still okay?" she heard Jesse asking, but it was as if his voice was coming from another planet. She tried to speak but wasn't sure it worked because all her energy was turned elsewhere. To her raging pussy. To the lines of ecstatic fire on her ass.

Unable to find her voice, she smiled and nodded.

He grinned back, evilly, then struck her again. This time the initial reaction was downright pain, and she yelped, but it transmuted to pleasure even as she cried out, spiraled deep inside her, seemed to reach her heart and soul.

"Another?"

She meant to say something truly deep along the lines of "Oh god, yes..." She didn't even get out that much, just a deep, throaty noise, but apparently Jesse understood.

He took her there. Gave her the pain. Not once, but three times in rapid succession, harder than the others. With the first two, she bit her lip, fought despite herself, despite feeling the pain transform itself almost immediately.

On the third, he ordered, "This time, come."

And she did.

They fucked after that, and somewhere along the line he untied her—maybe before or maybe in the middle, because at one point she was on top and couldn't have been if she were still tied that way—but her memory was foggy. Wave after wave of orgasm, and what felt like a serpent exploding up her spine, and Jesse's cock, Jesse's body, Jesse's beloved voice her only connection to the planet.

Afterward, when she could talk again, when the rest of the world coalesced around her again and she became aware of anything beyond the feel of Jesse, the scent of Jesse, the sound of Jesse, and later of her own vaguely aching muscles and tender ass, she turned to him and said, "Cheater."

"Whaa...?" He sounded about as vague as she felt.

"You didn't hit me anywhere near as hard as before."

"Yes, I did."

"But...but it was amazing. The other time just hurt."

He helped her stand, walked her over to the mirror, turned her around.

Her ass was a mottled mess, marked with seven distinct stripes.

"I...I..." She couldn't speak, just turned and buried her face in Jesse's chest.

"You're welcome," he said. "And thank you for trusting me to try again."

A noise somewhere between a sob and a laugh bubbled out of Heather. "Of course I trust you, Jesse," she whispered. "I know you. I love you. We both made mistakes that night, but we know what went wrong and we know better now. Thank you for believing me when I said I was ready to try again."

"Any time."

Heather stroked her tender ass and giggled. "I think we should wait a while before any more caning. But the oral sex when I was tied up...I could stand a little more of that."

Laughing, getting hard in anticipation, Jesse reached for the rope.

CHAPTER SEVEN

STAYING SAFE

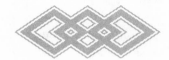

As someone who writes openly and honestly about sex, always using my own name and often including a photo of myself in things I publish, I often get emails and social media messages (and back when people still used such things—letters and phone messages) from anonymous strangers. Some of them are readers who want to say nice things (always awesome). Some of them are people who haven't read my work but want to remind me that I'm going to hell for writing about sex and that I should be ashamed of myself. (This used to be emotionally hard, but now that I'm older and wiser, they're easier to handle.) There's the large group of drive-by trolls—most of whom self-identify as male—who want me to write them back and tell them what wonderfully sexy things I'll do to them. (My usual response is, "Sure, I'd be happy to do that. I charge $1/word. Just send the money to PayPal and I'll write you a story." So far, no one has taken me up on it.)

And, finally, there are the people who are downright scary—who say they know who I am and where I live, and that they're coming after me. (Sometimes this is because I'm doing a "bad thing" by writing about sex, other times, their message has a sexual undertone to it, as though they think they know me because they read something that I wrote.)

I was telling a friend about this recently, and she said, "Why do you write under your own name, then? Why not use a pen name?"

There are a lot of answers to this—many of them having to do with my own belief the sex is not shameful and isn't something that I want to hide—but in this case the answer is because I believe I am safest when I am clearly visible and without secrets.

Case in point: A long time ago, I worked as a writer for a small-town newspaper during the day and was writing erotica—openly, as I never hid my sex-writing career from my employers—at night. I was also out as kinky and bisexual to anyone who asked. As part of my day job, I covered the PTA meetings of the nearby school. During one such meeting, one of the fathers on the PTA waited until I was in the middle of a large crowd, and then came up to me, pointed at me and said, very loudly, "You don't belong here, with our kids. You're an erotica writer. Now everyone knows that you write about sex!"

And I was able to look at him very calmly and say, "And now everyone knows that you read about it too."

I feel bad about shaming him that way—no one should be shamed by their interest in sex—but it was a protective, defensive measure, one that I was only able to take because I'd been open about my sexual interests and activities right out of the gate. When you have nothing to hide, it's really hard for other people to try to "out" you or shame you or uncover your "dirty little secrets." I'm open about who I am and what I do. I write about sex under my own name, I'll talk about my sexual interests and experiences to anyone who asks (even my own grandmother once, who delighted me with a question about where she could find my erotica books). But, that for me, IS my safety net. If everyone knows who I am and what I do, then there's no chance that someone can blindside me by attempting to use my "big secret" against me.

However, that's a choice that isn't for everyone. The effects on your children, career, family, religious affiliation and social interactions are important considerations. And in fact, I'm going to go the other direction entirely and suggest that you think very carefully about who you come out to and why. This isn't a statement of judgment or of being ashamed of who you are, but one of safety. Sadly, even today, there are people who view kinky activities as unhealthy, as signs of a depraved mind, body or spirit. These are people who might try to use your interests against you. Stories abound of bosses using BDSM interests as a reason to try and fire someone or of exes trying to get custody of children for the same reason.

Sharing information about your sexual interests, contact information, physical address and more on the Internet is common practice these days as well, whether it's on BDSM-specific sites or general websites and social media spaces. And there is no cap on how far information or photos like that can spread.

A good rule of thumb to remember is: once you put something out there—in writing, in photos, or even via dialogue—you can never take it back. Are you going to be okay with this person—and anyone that person might talk to or share something with—knowing this about you for the rest of your life?

On the other hand, paranoia or worrying about it too much can be detrimental to your emotional health. Try to find a balance between being careful and being afraid, and err on the side of caution if you feel at all nervous or concerned.

Get Your Passport Stamped: Safety Tips

1. Build a First Aid Kit

Author Jay Wiseman has a wonderful, comprehensive list of what to put in a first aid kit in his book, *Dungeon Emergencies and Supplies,* but you can start out with the basics: first, find a good container that can hold all of your stuff in one place, is leakproof and easy to clean and can be carried easily (if you move from place to place). Stock it with all the basics of a standard first aid kit, plus any safer sex items (condoms, dental dams, gloves, lube), instant heat/cold packs, a sharps container (if you're doing needle or blood play), any medications or inhalers, something to eat (in case of low blood sugar), and anything else that you might need.

If you use toys with locks, it's a good idea to keep extra keys in the emergency kit, as well as cutters that will quickly go through any fabric, leather, or metal cuffs, ties or chains that you plan on using. A final important, but often forgotten, element of any first aid kit is a well-charged cell phone, in case of emergencies.

2. Get to Know the Nearest Hospital

It's the kind of thing you hope you will never have to use, but if you're planning to practice kinky sex, learn the location of and quickest route to the nearest emergency room. Hospitals are scary enough in any emergency, without the added pressure of it being sexual in nature. In some places, health workers are trained in (or at least open-minded about) sex injuries, but in others, you may face sarcasm, judgment, ridicule or ignorance. None of that matters. You (or your partner) need and deserve medical treatment. Don't avoid the hospital due to shame or fear. Don't lie about why you're there. (You're not going to fool the doctors and nurses anyway, and the best way to get help is to be clear and honest about what happened.)

If you're not the one who is injured, be the other person's advocate and protector. Don't abandon him or her, be very clear with the staff that this was consensual sex where something went wrong, and if you feel like someone might report it as assault, call your kink-positive lawyer right away.

3. Know the Law

Believe it or not, BDSM is still considered to be illegal in a number of places. This means that even when the activities are clearly consensual, kinky sex can be prosecuted under state criminal laws, specifically those that deal with aggravated assault, sexual assault and sexual abuse. While these laws are important, as they protect those who are violated or harmed against their will, they can also be used to incorrectly criminalize activities that are clearly consensual.

The general rule in most places is that a criminal act occurs when one personal causes another person physical harm. The law doesn't see two adults engaging in mutually agreed upon actions; it just sees one person causing harm to another. Thus, BDSM isn't typically treated as sex act; it's treated as a violent act.

Add to that the general cultural misunderstanding of kinky sex, and you have a criminal system that's ripe for confusion. The most common ways in which criminal prosecution can occur around kinky sex are: when a BDSM experience turns out to be more intense, painful or damaging than the submissive partner expected or wanted, and he or she goes to the police; if a partner in a BDSM scene requires medical attention and is reported to the authorities by hospital personnel, an observer, or a friend or relative; or when a BDSM relationship ends badly, and the submissive partner files charges of assault or abuse.

This is just one reason why explicit, informed consent is so important. Protect yourself and your partners by knowing the law in your area, and by making it clear that everything you're doing is something that you've both agreed to.

4. Vet Your New Partners

Be very careful when meeting or playing with a new partner, especially the first time. Common sense is the key here. Meet in a public place. It isn't wise to let someone tie you up or otherwise restrain you (especially if the two of you are alone) the first time you meet him. Line up a "safe call"—a friend who is waiting for your phone calls or texts (in which you're supposed to use a specific code word) at specific times throughout your meeting and who has all of the information about who you are with and where you're going. I also recommend telling the person that you're with that you've lined up a safe call (without giving away the details). Anyone who has your best interests in mind will be glad that you're being safe; if someone reacts poorly to the idea of a safe call, then it's a good idea to walk away.

You might also try bsafe (getbsafe.com), a free personal safety app for your phone that allows you to quickly and easily stay safe and connected.

BE PREPARED:

Jay Wiseman on Handling Emergencies

Jay Wiseman is an author, video producer, presenter, workshop leader, activist and expert witness.

You have an unusual vantage point on safety within the kink world, based upon your experience as an EMS worker and as a former law school professor. Can you talk a little bit about what you've learned from your unique perspective?

I think the main way my eight years of doing ambulance work has affected my view of BDSM is that the possibility that "something could go wrong" is much less abstract for me. It's one thing to know that drunk drivers can cause auto accidents. It's quite another thing to be called to the scene of seven such accidents over the course of a three-day weekend. When you get called to an accident scene in which some drunk has gone over the center line and shattered a family of five completely innocent people, that sort of thing stays with you.

This applies to my view of BDSM. In contemplating what could go wrong, it's less abstract for me than it is for many other people. I can imagine the resulting horror. Fortunately, it's fairly easy to mitigate the major risks.

As to my legal training, it allows me to foresee the legal consequences of what might happen if things go seriously wrong in a way that a person not particularly educated in law cannot foresee. For instance, there's no right to a free attorney if you're sued. You'll pay for one out of your own pocket, and if you can't afford one then you're really in trouble. Also, it improves one's understanding of matters such as the fact that there's no consent defense for very reckless forms of BDSM play such as gun play, so if a scene like that goes wrong, the top is seriously in trouble.

What is the most important bit of safety advice that you would give to everyone who's exploring BDSM?

Two things: First, take your time. There's no rush to do any of this, and particularly there's no rush to do BDSM with a particular person. Take your time to really get to know the other person and establish that he or she is a trustworthy person. I really like the definition of trust that I read in a novel years ago: trust is the residue of kept agreements.

Second, get your information from a variety of sources. There is no one true, holy-grail source of BDSM information. That said, experienced players generally agree on the major points. If a would-be teacher is offering instruction that is very different from how a particular topic usually gets taught, then that would-be teacher has the burden of explaining why he or she takes an alternative approach.

If every kinky person was going to get some basic medical training, what would you recommend they learn?

I'd recommend a one-day class in basic CPR and first aid, repeated at least every two years. If possible, try to get this training from someone with significant field experience in actually providing such care. I've found a lot of truth in the saying that, "Amateurs teach amateurs how to be amateurs." Try to get training from a pro. I've taught First Aid/ CPR classes for more than forty years, and I can walk into another instructor's class and in five minutes tell you how much actual experience they do or don't have.

THE ONLY REAL GIRL
ON THE INTERNET

Stella Harris

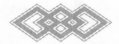

I poured hot wax all over my tits and gave a dildo an enthusiastic blow job and titty fuck." Shelly started choking on her muffin before Lisa even finished answering her. That would teach her not to ask about Lisa's late-night exploits while she was eating.

When Shelly recovered from her near-death experience—no Heimlich maneuver required—she stared at Lisa in wide-eyed horror, her mouth gaping like a fish's.

"What?" Lisa asked, starting to feel self-conscious. She usually told Shelly everything, but maybe it was time to keep some secrets.

"I'd like to think I didn't hear you right, but I don't want to risk you saying it again." Shelly fortified herself with a large gulp of coffee before she spoke again. "I don't understand why you do this stuff," she finally said, after seeming to abandon several other statements.

"Because he asked me to," Lisa answered with the simple truth.

Shelly didn't seem to understand the magnitude of responsibility Lisa felt about being the only real girl on the Internet. All those lonely men out there, cocks in hand, just waiting for someone to get them off. It was a big job, but someone had to do it. And Lisa had to admit she got a thrill from it. Watching a guy blow his load because of her was the ultimate power trip and she couldn't get enough.

It didn't matter what the guy looked like—and sometimes she couldn't even see their faces—all that mattered was that they were counting on her. The way their faces lit up when they saw her, or the frantic typing begging her not to leave, was a heady rush.

Plus, she could follow her fantasies, completely let herself go, in the safety of her own home. She never gave out her real name or details about herself. It was safe, sexy fun with strangers, the kind she could never have in real life.

Lisa didn't think of herself as most guys' wet dream. Men flirted with her, sometimes, but no one she met on the street coveted her the way the men in the chatrooms did at night, when she became their whole world. They called her "pretty" or "beautiful" or "sexy" and she even thought they meant it, at least in the moment.

Whether they begged or demanded, they all wanted something from her, and it was in her power to grant or deny their requests. Up to her to decide if they got off quickly, aroused beyond their expectations by someone actually fulfilling their requests, or whether they were left hanging, trying to find a willing partner until their patience ran out or they had to make do with whatever low-quality free porn they could scrounge from an Internet search.

"My living room looks like a scene from a frat party, and I was home alone. I'm still finding wax in places you don't want to hear about." Shelly grimaced, putting the horror she felt at what Lisa was saying into one sour expression.

"It's like when you go to the beach and end up finding sand everywhere for days," Lisa continued, blatantly ignoring Shelly's distaste at the subject matter. "You could join me sometime, if you wanted; I bet half the guys would come untouched at the sight of two girls on the screen," Lisa teased, earning a muffin crumb flicked in her direction.

"Not a chance in hell. I want no part of your perverse hobby," Shelly said emphatically, wrinkling her nose as if the very idea reeked.

Lisa wasn't sure why she kept telling Shelly these stories. She obviously didn't enjoy them, even if she did get the occasional shocked, tell-me-more look on her face. Lisa supposed she just needed to share with at least one person to make it real. Well, at least one person from her offline life.

Each time a blank screen popped up, it was the start of a new adventure. *You are now talking to a stranger. Say hello.*

These men thought they were in control, that they were getting what they wanted. But really they were letting Lisa see them in their most vulnerable state. There was something utterly primal about it, and Lisa had a visceral reaction to every hard cock exposed to her. Whether it was already on display when the screen came on or only revealed later, her mouth would water, her cunt would throb or her ass would ache. She wanted each and every one of those cocks.

Another night found Lisa firing up her laptop—glass of wine in hand, candles lit around the room. It was go time.

You are now talking to a stranger. Say hello.

Lisa smiled at the screen as her stranger came into view: a good-looking man in his mid-to-late twenties with short blond hair and a bit of blond scruff, and musical instruments visible in the background.

He leaned forward, squinted at the screen and smiled when he saw her. He had a nice smile and her own expression brightened in response. *Hi* appeared on her screen.

Hi there she typed, keeping her eyes on his image. He was shirtless, just wearing what looked like pajama pants, and it was dim in the room. She wondered if he was in her time zone.

What are you doing tonight? He was starting slow, being polite. Lisa appreciated the effort, but she didn't need to be wooed. She was eager to see what the rest of this man looked like.

Just killing time. She'd tried a number of responses to this common question, and ultimately found it worked best to let the guys think they were talking her into doing something out of character. She'd tried answering *hoping to see your cock* once and her stranger disconnected. Men are so easily frightened off.

Cool.

What are you looking for tonight? she prompted. He smiled and looked away; he might even have blushed—it was too dark to tell.

Don't be shy, she added.

Can I see your breasts? There, that was more like it. She waited a moment, not wanting to seem too eager. Slowly, she pulled her shirt down beneath her breasts—she'd learned early on to wear something loose and low-cut enough to pull off this maneuver. It looked more realistic than just whipping off her shirt at the first request.

Her one-man audience watched avidly, leaning toward the screen, his hands twitching on his knees. She paused, as if considering whether she should go farther, and then pulled her bra aside as well. He leaned forward to get a better look at her breasts as they spilled out. She crossed her arms beneath them for support, showing them to their best advantage. She loved her breasts and watching him look at her was already getting her wet.

Can you play with them? He was getting more comfortable now that it was clear she was game, but she wasn't that easy.

What about you? He must have been waiting for the prompt, because he stood immediately and dropped his pants. He was even better looking than she'd first realized. A light smattering of hair on his chest led to smooth, firm abs. As her eyes wandered lower, she saw that he was fully hard already, and his erection stood out from his body as he showed off for the camera before sitting down again.

She smiled at him, typed *nice* and began to stroke her breasts. He watched her for a moment before letting a hand fall to his cock. His eyes never left the screen as he began stroking off and Lisa did her best to put on a good show. Clearly he was a boob man, as he wasn't asking for more.

He stared, entranced as Lisa stroked her tits, pinched and even licked her own nipples. He remained riveted to the screen as his hand moved faster on his cock, his free hand clutching at his knee rhythmically—perhaps fantasizing about feeling Lisa up.

She imagined that hand touching her, stroking her breasts, reaching lower, those long fingers slipping into her wet cunt. She considered writing these things to him, but he seemed so focused she kept the fantasy to herself.

Lisa watched as he continued to beat off, imagined him thrusting into her instead of into his own hand. She watched as his face contorted with pleasure and he spilled over his hand and began moving slower. She sat back from the screen, covered herself and smiled.

That was awesome, thank you. She always appreciated the gratitude and he seemed genuinely pleased.

You're welcome, she typed, wondering how long they'd make small talk. It wasn't long, it turned out, before he bid her good night.

The screen went dark, the countdown began, and in five seconds she was connected to the next stranger; another man, younger than the first. His face lit up with a bright smile at the sight of her and she wondered how long he'd been online, just waiting for someone to talk to. *How old are you?* she typed, just to be sure.

24. His response was immediate. He would be easy to please, she could tell already. He still looked at her—or the image of her on his screen—like he couldn't believe she was real.

What's your name? She thought for a moment. She didn't usually give her real name, not that it mattered. She could see light coming through his windows; he was on the other side of the world.

Lisa. He smiled again, a lightning-fast flash of bright white teeth.

I don't date much, I'm not good with girls... he wrote and looked at the screen, his face contorting with what had to be nerves—or fear of rejection.

That's okay, just tell me what you like.

Do you have a candle? So this was how things were going to go, she thought, holding up one of the votives from the table in answer.

Pour wax on your tits. Nerves put aside, he got right down to business. She'd done this before and knew it would hurt. She couldn't help but hesitate before she removed her top and bra.

It's going to be very hot.

Pour from higher up. Hm. He'd done this before, too. She held the candle a good ten inches above her chest and began to tilt it slightly, not wanting too much wax at once. She watched as a stream flowed from the candle and splashed across her breast. She saw it hit her skin, but it was another moment before she felt it. A hot sting that ached as it sunk in. It took all her willpower not to brush the wax away and soothe her flesh.

The words *Good girl* appeared on her screen and she smiled. This was what he wanted. *Do the other one.* Lisa moved the candle above her other breast and tilted it even more slowly—she knew how much it was going to hurt now and it made her hesitate.

Position after position, she followed his orders: spilling hot wax on her breasts, ass, thighs, stomach and pussy. Whatever he asked for she did and his praise was addictive. Wax wasn't really her thing, but watching him get off on it absolutely was. She hoped he'd ask for something that would get her off, too. But she was always surprised by how few guys actually wanted to watch her have an orgasm.

He was stroking himself furiously now; she couldn't believe he was lasting this long. She'd never seen a guy his age with this kind of stamina. *I want to see you stick something in your ass.* She wasn't sure if she should laugh or not. The frankness with which he made his requests was astounding. She was less experienced in this area but wanted to please him.

Hang on, she typed, before dashing out of the room to check her nightstand. She eyed her selection of toys critically. She didn't have many toys made for ass play and so her choices were more limited than she would have liked. But she didn't want to disappoint her young friend. She grabbed a toy with a wide, flared base and hurried back to her laptop. She held the toy up in front of the screen and awaited his approval.

The response was immediate. *Perfect. Put it in.*

Lisa took a quick moment offscreen to lube the toy and then positioned herself so that her ass would be in view. Not really an easy task, especially as she tried to watch the screen for further praise or commands.

As she slid the toy into her ass she was surprised to find how easily it accommodated the intrusion, at least for the first few inches.

More, the screen prompted her. She took a deep breath and pushed. It started to hurt and she paused to let her muscles relax before pushing farther. She could see her boy leaning toward his screen, mouth open in pleasure as his hand flew on his cock.

This is the best thing that ever happened to me. She saw the words on the screen but didn't stop what she was doing.

Burning tits, a pounding ass, and a boy that loves you. Her heart thudded at the admission; she smiled and cringed at once. This wasn't love, not even close. She didn't believe in love at first sight, only lust. But he was young. She didn't respond.

Tell me that you love me.

I can't do that, baby. She wouldn't lie. It wouldn't be fair to either of them. Leave it to her to find the one guy online that wanted more than a quick orgasm. He was so earnest it was heartbreaking.

This was a one-time thing; it had to be. She was the only real girl on the Internet, and countless other men were waiting their turn.

CHAPTER EIGHT

HANDLING ROUGH TERRAIN

W hen I was in my late thirties, I was diagnosed with Lyme disease. In case you've never heard of it, Lyme is an infectious disease caused by ticks. It's not well understood, but it can have long-term symptoms like joint paint, flu-like aching around the joints, numbness and weakness in the limbs and impaired muscle movement. Basically: it is the suck. For months, I could barely get out of bed, I was pumped full of antibiotics and I was in so much pain that I couldn't even type words into my computer.

Not surprisingly, during that time my sex life went out the window. Feeling like I was dying wasn't conducive to any kind of sexiness. Thankfully, I eventually started feeling better. I was still on antibiotics, but I was able to get out of bed a few hours a day and start moving around. Along with some sense of wellness and a profound sense of gratitude that I was still alive, I found that my mind starting turning, bit by bit, to pleasures. Food sounded good again. I was ready to start writing once more. And sexual pleasure; my mind turned to sexual pleasure most of all. I wanted to stop fighting my body and be its friend again. I wanted to find something positive in the curves of my skin, to no longer feel like my body was betraying me. I wanted a fantastic, mind-blowing orgasm so I could forget about how awful I felt, if only for a few minutes.

Unfortunately, while my mind was all about pleasures, no one told my body that it was time to move in that direction. I threw up most food that had any flavor. My finger joints were stiff and sore after writing just a few sentences. And whether due to the illness or the anti-biotics, I found that sexual pleasure had become an elusive, slippery thing. Masturbating or even holding a vibrator made my wrists ache. I couldn't have an orgasm. I couldn't stand the thought of someone else touching me, because I was afraid of the possible pain. And that brought up all kinds of other issues—if I was so afraid of pain, what did that mean for the future of my kinky sex life? I started worrying that the illness (or its cure) had permanently damaged me, that my life would be empty of sexual pleasure forever.

Thankfully, that wasn't the case. My body—and my mental state—returned to a place where I could enjoy sex, even dirty, kinky sex, once again. Even after more than five years of being symptom free, I will never forget that experience, trying to wade my way back to sexual pleasure through the murky swamp of illness and depression.

In a perfect world, every bit of sex in our lives would be about plea-sure and joy. But as we all know, all too often, life interferes with those plans. Our mental and physical health, cultural and family pressures, grief, stress…all of these things can have huge impacts on our sex lives no matter where we fall on the kinky spectrum. They don't have to be huge roadblocks on your kinky journey, though. A little planning and understanding of the possible potholes means that you can get past them and get on your way to kinky pleasure in no time.

Potholes on the Pleasure Trail

Illness: Short-term illnesses, like a cold or a broken wrist, probably don't add too much stress to a sexual relationship. Both partners know that the change is temporary, and with everyone focused on healing the person who's unwell, there's probably not a lot of worry about sex over the long haul. Still, finding new ways to express your desire and arousal while you're healing keeps the fire alive, and helps make sure you're ready to jump back into bed with fervor when you're feeling better.

Long-term, chronic or terminal illnesses, however, can be something else entirely. Having sex during those times is hard enough, but what about when you and your partner have a sex life built on giving each other pain, on tying each other up, or spending long hours on your knees, waiting patiently for your reward? If your partner is sick, weak or hurting, it's hard to know how to respond. Does your partner have the stamina to dominate you like he used to? If your partner used to love being brought to tears with biting and spanking, but now is dealing with chronic aches, does pain no longer appeal to him sexually? These are questions that only you and your partner can answer.

As with all other elements of sex, communication is the key. Not just with each other, but with the health-care professionals in your life. Patience, understanding and a willingness to give your partner what he or she wants and needs can take the pressure off you both.

Aging: In our culture, sexy equals young. Or at least that's what the advertisements and marketing would have you believe. As we get older, our bodies change in ways that we may not expect, but that in itself shouldn't be a deterrent to having a fulfilling sex life. In fact, when you start looking at the figures, it turns out that huge numbers of seniors are enjoying sex—and kinky sex in particular. Now that they are retired and their kids are grown and off doing their own thing, many older people have the time and freedom to explore their sexual interests in ways they couldn't before.

Some general things to be aware of as we age are joint issues, circulation concerns and thinning skin. Our senses can begin to dull as we grow older as well, so it's important to adjust our forms of consent and ways of checking in with each other. As we start to lose our hearing or our vision, safewords need to become hand signals, while visible actions may need to transform to something auditory. Erectile dysfunction, lack of self-lubrication, and decreased sensitivity could also be concerns. However, for the most part, aging is just another change that we go through, like our sexual identity. With proper communication and awareness, it's one that's rife with exploration, discovery and pleasure.

Feminism and BDSM: I once saw a poster that read EVERY TIME MY BOYFRIEND SPANKS ME, MY INNER FEMINIST WEEPS. BUT IT JUST FEELS SO DAMN GOOD. As an avid kinkster and a fierce advocate for gender rights, I found that reading that poster was what made *my* inner feminist weep.

It's true that feminism and BDSM have long been at odds with each other. One adage goes that you can't be a fierce, independent woman if you want to be spanked, bound or dominated (especially not if it's by a man). Others argue that women who want to be submissive to a man are just acting out patriarchal fantasies, have been coerced into thinking this is something that they want, or that they're just unknowingly perpetuating and supporting violence against women.

And it's not just women—men who bottom are seen as less-than, as though they are somehow betraying their gender by not wanting to be the dominant one. Men who top are sometimes labeled misogynistic or sexist.

While I can't speak for everyone, I will argue that for the vast majority of women, those arguments are bullshit. Safe, sane, and consensual pleasure is an expression of power, freedom and individuality no matter how you define your gender. No one else gets to tell you what's right for you, what gives you pleasure or how your sexual identity interacts with your other identities. If it feels right for you and your partner, then it's right for your feminism (or whatever label you claim as your own).

Rape and Ravishment Fantasies: One last thing that I want to talk about in this section concerns our deepest, darkest secrets. Those fantasies that we hide away in the back corners of our brains because something deep inside us tells us that they're not okay. Some of the most common of these are fantasies that involve abduction, ravishment, forced activities and rape. People of all genders, sexual orientations and interests have these kinds of fantasies, and most of us are taught there's something horribly wrong with us if we even entertain such desires. But studies show again and again that fantasies like this are common among both men and women. Some people who have rape fantasies have experienced actual traumatic sexual events in their lives, and others haven't.

The important thing to remember is that not only are fantasies like this normal and common, they're also just that—fantasies. Something that allows us to push the boundaries in a safe place, usually in our imaginations or in secure environments with sane, safe, trusted, consenting adults. The distinction between fantasy and reality is very clear—while there might be the illusion of nonconsensuality in fantasies or fantasy reenactments like these, everything is actually carefully negotiated beforehand, including limits, safewords, emotional touchstones and expectations.

A final word of caution: if you are role-playing consensual nonconsensuality, it's a good idea to create a signed, physical contract as evidence of the agreement between the two partners. This way you're both protected, and you don't have to worry about anyone misunderstanding the experience.

Get Your Passport Stamped: Hang Tough

1. Get Out of Your Body.

If you or your partner is dealing with a short- or long-term illness that makes physical contact difficult, try having mental sex instead. Read each other erotic stories, listen to erotic audio books, watch sexy movies or just tell your partner how much you lust after him. Turning tools of torture into tools of soft touch—using a flogger as a gentle massager, for example—is another way to remind your partner of what you still share and of what your future holds, without asking anything of him that he can't give.

2. Give When You Can.

During times of grief, sadness, illness or other emotional or physical difficulty, your partner may not have the energy to engage with you on a physical level. Offer to do the work in the form of a hand job, a light spanking, a vibratory climax or anything else that will make your partner feel good without having to exert energy.

If you are the partner struggling, make the effort to connect with your partner when your energy is high, even if it's just to make out for a few minutes. It reminds your loved one that you see him or her as more than just a caregiver, and gives you both a chance to connect when you're feeling your best.

3. Explore Your Darkest Fantasies

If you have fantasies that you've never really admitted (perhaps not even to yourself), start exploring them in a way that feels safe and comfortable. Daydream for a few minutes before you fall asleep. Start a fantasy journal, where you give yourself permission to explore your interests. If you have a partner who you feel safe with, begin to talk to her about your desires, and see where it takes you. You may find that you're not the only one who is craving ravishment—and exploring this type of fantasy together can take your sexual experiences to incredible new places.

FICTION

THE WRONG WOMAN

Kristina Lloyd

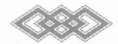

S omeone had fucked up," went the story. He was supposed to be handsome and charming, and they should have been in a restaurant playing footsie under the table while a waiter took their order, glass and cutlery tinkling around them.

Instead, Jody was in a dingy alley with a gun to her back, her hair awry, her stockings laddered. "Keep walking," he said. "Look straight ahead."

Her legs were shaking. That wasn't in the story. Cobbles rippled like water in the pale-white sheen of a streetlight and, in her heels, she struggled on the uneven terrain like a weak-limbed foal.

"You've got the wrong woman." Her throat was dry, her voice a rasp.

"Don't get cute," he said. "Here. Left here. I've got some friends who want to meet you."

Around the corner, he made her stand by a broad wooden door as he tied her hands behind her back, looping rope around her wrists in a figure eight. Brittle strips of green paint hung like lolling tongues from the wood and six small, high windows suggested a dirty, cobwebbed interior. When Jody's hands were secured, the man heaved on a handle to roll the doors aside, the scene opening up as it might in a theater when the curtains were raised. Before them was a cobble-floored car-repair garage, its ceiling veiled by a sagging pigeon net from which crisp, brown ivy dangled like vines in a ghostly rainforest. The light was dim and the props, if you could call them that, were scanty: a heap of old tires, two rusty cars at the rear, an armchair sprouting stuffing and various tools scattered randomly about the place. No one was in sight.

Her heels echoed on the cobbles as they walked into the center of the garage, and she imagined the knocking of her heart was equally loud. She breathed in smells of damp, dust, oil and scorched metal. She didn't know if the gun at her back was real but it didn't matter. If you thought it might be, it was.

One by one, they emerged from the shadows, five muscular men in jeans and vests, all bristling with menace and swagger. They crowded around her and she was on her knees before she knew it, the cobbles harsh and cold. The blouse she'd worn for her restaurant date tore easily. A pair of clumsy hands shoved the ripped silk around her shoulders while more hands scooped her breasts from her bra and twisted her nipples. She writhed and squealed in protest.

"You've got the wrong woman," she said again, but they only laughed.

One of the men unzipped. She looked up at her circle of tormentors and that's when her world really began to spin. Dizziness turned to blackness before her vision stabilized and the colors returned. She knew him, the guy with his cock out who was glowering down at her. She knew him.

He clearly recognized her too. He edged closer.

"I knew this was a bad idea," he said. The end of his cock butted at her lips. "So let's make it a good one."

She refused to open for him. He pinched her jaw in his big hand, forcing her lips apart. "Devious little bitch. That's right, open up." As he slid into her mouth, he softly added, "There you go, Jody."

How the hell did she know him? She wracked her brains but her thoughts were stalled when another pair of hands went rummaging under her skirt.

"Let's see how much she likes it, eh?"

"Who gives a fuck whether she likes it or not?"

Her body betrayed her secret, her wetness slicking onto unknown, probing fingers.

"Hey, pay attention, lady. You got another dick here."

"And here."

More unzipping, more swollen, ruddy-tipped cocks bobbing around her, zips splayed like teeth. She moved from the first cock to another belonging to a guy who soon withdrew to give one of his mates access to her ready mouth. The third guy was rough and forceful, the end of his cock bumping at her throat, making her gag and splutter. Tears and saliva spilled down her face.

"Take it," he warned, lodging himself deep.

Her tethered hands unbalanced her, but she was steadied by a fist clutching a clump of hair so hard it pinched her scalp. It was the guy who knew her name. His knowledge felt more dangerous than the gun.

They all fucked her mouth. At one point they made her take two cocks simultaneously, her lips stretched wide to accommodate both lengths. It was ungainly, awkward and physically unsatisfying for her and presumably them. But the psychological aspect was para-mount, their triumphalism in her humiliation mattering more than the pleasure derived from a snug, slippery grip.

Eventually they started to come, almost as a single entity. One guy spurting into her mouth prompted another guy to jerk off onto her breasts, his groans of bliss prompting another to take himself in hand while a fourth ordered her to open her mouth, making her a receptacle for his aim.

When the guy who knew her name climaxed, she heard him roar, saw how his face flushed and the way the sinews in his neck popped out, tight and hard as guitar strings beneath his skin.

"Yes!" he hissed, throwing back his head.

Finally, she remembered who he was, remembered seeing that raw, animal passion as the man, ecstatic, had fallen to his knees. Her blood ran cold.

The feedback form was lengthy. But, said the agency, post-scene data collection was vital for their continued provision of satisfactory fantasy fulfillment.

Did the experience meet your expectations? Prefer not to answer.

Did you feel safe? Yes. No.

Did you find the men/women attractive? Yes.

Did you climax? No.

Will you climax, or have you climaxed, by recalling the scenario afterward? Prefer not to answer.

Any other comments? You got the wrong woman. I didn't ask for this. I recognized one of the men. He plays five-a-side with my husband on the first Sunday of every month at Lowfell Park. My husband must never, ever find out. Please tell that man it was a mistake. Tell him not to tell my husband. Tell him you got the wrong woman, and I might sue. Tell him someone fucked up. I didn't ask to be used and degraded by a bunch of thugs in some squalid garage. I didn't ask to be tied up and have cock after cock

thrust into my mouth. You got the wrong woman. Tell him.
Would you use our agency again? Yes.
If so, what sort of fantasy scenario might you like us to arrange? The
wrong woman fantasy.

FICTION

THE SUN IS AN ORDINARY STAR

Shanna Germain

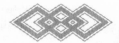

He was cleaning the bedroom for Stella's return when he heard it. He'd been down on his haunches, swishing the broom beneath the bed's dark corners when something metallic clanked against the broom. He fished it out.

There, among the dust bunnies and dirt, was Stella's favorite set of nipple clamps, two silver clips connected by a thin chain. The metal was dusty and a few of Stella's long hairs were wound in the chain. Still on his haunches, he picked the clamps up. They were lighter than he remembered, more fragile, the weight of them in his palm almost nothing.

He opened one of the large clips, ran his finger across the row of teeth. Croc heads, Stella called them. Before everything, she'd call home from the office some days, leave a message on the machine. "You're going to have to get out the crocs tonight," she'd say.

Last time she'd called home was right before Christmas. She'd been working on the big holiday shoe campaign, photo-shopping sweat and muscles and boobs onto famous athletes. Even on the message her voice was shaky. "Baby, I am not feeling up to par," she said. "Let's get those alligator maws out tonight. And whatever else you can think of. I know you're gonna make me feel better."

And he had. As soon as she'd walked in the door, still in her cream-colored work pants and the brown blouse that matched her eyes, her long dark hair pulled back, he'd ordered her to undress. She looked tired, light-gray circles under her big brown eyes, but she'd asked and he always tried to give her what she asked for. He'd ordered her to undress him too, and then he'd cuffed her arms to their slatted head-board. She was pale curves against the purple bedspread. Her long hair, loose from its clip, waved out around her head.

With her arms above her head, her small tits tilted upward. He loved her tits, pale and down-fuzzed as summer peaches, but it was her nipples that he loved the most, the way they stretched high and taut when she was aroused. He'd teased her first, rubbing the sharp edge of the clamp teeth along the inside of her thigh, around the edges of her neck, in smaller and smaller circles around her nipples. He loved to watch the points push into her skin.

Stella was as still as he'd told her to be, mouth closed, only her flared nostrils giving away her arousal. When he saw she was wet, he slid the opened clamp along the edge of her pussy lips, up to her clit. He'd never clamped her there, but he'd promised her it was coming. Now he closed the clamp, just a bit, on that pale pink flesh. She arched her back and gasped.

He took the clamps away, slapped the curvy bottom of her ass, hard enough to feel the sting on his palm. "Be still," he said.

She closed her eyes, her nostrils flaring. When her eyes were closed, he opened both clamps and then closed them on the rosy skin of her nipples. Stella inhaled deeply through her nose.

He leaned back and watched her, the metal clips closed onto her taut flesh, leaving little pinpoints of bloodless skin. At the end of the bed, Stella's feet, the only thing she couldn't keep still, arched in their bonds. Her clit was aching, he knew. "You want to be fucked?" he asked.

Stella knew enough to keep quiet, even to shake her head a little from side to side.

He put one finger inside the hot, wetness of her, curled it into an arch. "No?" he asked.

"No," she said. But her pussy gave her away, the way she stretched against her bonds to take more of his finger inside her. He entered her with a second finger.

"You're sure?" he asked. He loved to watch her at this moment. His Stella, stubborn as her Aries sign, truth speaking, type A. The internal struggle—to say what she wanted, to take what she wanted, or to give in, just for these few moments, to him. This, he knew, was why she wanted to be topped, needed to be topped. This was why he loved it. His cock loved it too, of course, but his mind loved to get her here, to this final release.

He wiggled his fingers inside her, hard against her walls. "I'm sorry, what?" he said, even though she hadn't said anything.

"No," she breathed. Just once. But he knew it was enough. He took his fingers out. "Look at me," he said. And she did, while he entered her, his cock going deep inside her and one hand pulling the nipple clamps, hard and harder, until she begged to be let loose.

He reached up and unbuckled the cuffs. "One hand on your clit." She did as he said; she put one hand on her clit, two fingers rubbing furiously back and forth. It was almost enough to make him come, the sight of her.

He entered her again, keeping himself back far enough that she could still work her clit. Her other hand reached for something to hold onto. "The clamps," he said. "Pull."

And she did, pulling her nipples up and up with the chain, arching her back to press her clit into him and her hand. He came before she did but was hard enough to keep inside until she came. Her orgasm was soft, quiet moans and one last tug on the clamps.

He eased himself out of her and sat beside her on the bed. When he took the clamps from her nipples, she moaned again, turning her head away. He kissed her nipples gently. She turned back toward him, her brown eyes no longer squinted-up from stress. She still looked tired though, beneath her eyes and around the edges of her lips. He stroked her hair and she snuggled her face into the curve of his neck. "You always know just what I need," she said. And then she'd fallen asleep, her breath soft and quiet against his skin.

That was six weeks, two surgeries and some kind of new-fangled chemo ago. Today, Stella was coming home. He didn't know what to do with the clamps, and he couldn't bear to touch the cold metal any longer, so he opened the nightstand drawer.

The books from friends and family—*Coping with Cancer, Outsmart Your Cancer, Cancer Husband*—stared up at him, spines uncracked. He'd tried to read the *Husband* one during one of Stella's appointments, but he hadn't understood what was about to happen, and the chapters on lumpectomy and chemo and sex with cancer had seemed impossible. Now, he wished he'd read it, at least the sex chapter, although he doubted there was anything about the kind of sex he and Stella had. Used to have. They'd had sex once or twice while she was sick, but it had been the kind of soft, gentle sex he'd always imagined belonged to virgins and old people. When Stella's bones hurt after hot showers and she couldn't sleep because the sheets tore at her skin, they'd fallen into this habit of moving quietly together, him raising himself above her, cock and pussy the only place they touched. And then even that had fallen away, forgotten under the bed in the midst of doctors and options and books and Stella's determination.

Stella had tackled cancer the same way she tackled a big project at work, or when he'd first met her, a research paper in grad school. Learn the facts, make a to-do list, and then checkmark your way down to the end. Get diagnosed, check. Find the best doctor they could afford, check. Explore all the treatments, check. Get rid of it, check. He didn't want to admit it, but Stella had handled this all with her usual grace and determination, while he was the one who felt lost.

Now, they had cut it out of her body, and she was coming home to him. And he felt like the world's biggest asshole for what he wanted. Or the world's whiniest kid: my wife went to Cancerville and all I got was this stupid T-shirt. He wanted her down on her knees, the gorgeous globes of her ass pink-marked, begging him for mercy. He wanted to tie her and enter her, one half-inch at a time, until she bucked her hips against him. He wanted to clamp the clips in his hand around the points of her nipples and force her to fuck herself until she came, until the tightness left her body and she could fall asleep again, at the point of his neck, without worry. He wanted to give her that release, but without topping her, without hurting a body that had already been beaten by its own cells, he didn't know how.

Just the possibility of it made his cock harden. He reached down to rub himself through his pants, and then he realized he was still holding the nipple clamps. Shiny guilt-makers. He dropped them onto the pile of books and shut the drawer tight. It was almost time to pick Stella up anyway.

Stella came home from the hospital with a new pair of glasses and a new star, dark red against her pale skin. He saw the glasses as soon as she got in the car—she put the blue- and yellow-striped frames on so she could see the street signs, even though she wasn't driving. He hadn't seen the star yet, but he felt it radiating from her body, sending heat through her white T-shirt, through the blue fleece she wore over it, through the shawl she had wrapped around her shoulders. The heat made him feel like he'd just landed on the surface of some unknown sun. Sweat started at the edges of his hairline.

In the seat beside him, Stella shivered. He took his hand off the window button.

"Temperature okay?" he asked. She turned from the window. Her now-short hair was peppered with early gray above her ears. The pinkish tint of the glasses turned her brown eyes toward black, made the purple half-moons beneath her eyes even darker.

"It's fine," Stella said. "Thank you."

Her voice sounded like a grandmother's, soft and sugar-sweet. In fact, everything about her screamed grandmother: the half-sized glasses, the way she held onto the seat belt with one bird-bone hand, the slow sighs that she didn't even know she was making. Still, she held herself straight up in her seat, not allowing her head to lean on the seat rest.

"Your mom bring the glasses?" he asked, to hear her speak instead of sigh.

Stella touched the earpiece as though she'd forgotten she had them on. "I rang a nurse," she said. She took the glasses off and folded them. "Had them brought up from the gift shop. My vision's gone haywire."

Stella had her head back at the window. He watched her while he drove. The disease had tightened her round face, made her cheekbones seem higher and larger. His instinct was to reach between the seats and take her hand. Reassure her: they got it all, everything's fine. But he couldn't stand to see her turn back toward him, to see her eyes hidden behind the lenses.

She surprised him by reaching her hand out to his across the space. He took it, even though he needed to shift. He didn't understand

much about what was happening or why, but he understood that you
didn't waste time and you didn't turn down an extended hand. Her
hand felt light and empty, a discarded crab shell.

With her other hand, Stella rubbed at something on the window.
"I'm tired," she said. It seemed to be the beginning of a sentence. He
waited, her hand lighter and lighter in his own. The only sound was
the rev of the unshifted car and the squeak of Stella's finger against
the window. These sounds stretched out so long he thought he might
have misjudged, maybe there wasn't more she wanted to say. He let his
foot farther off the gas—they were going twenty in a forty now—and
opened his mouth.

Stella tightened her fingers on his. "I'm tired," she said again. "But
I was thinking..." she broke off, rubbed the window harder. A car
came up behind them, blinked its lights. He shifted the wheel to the
right, gave them space to go around. His ears felt like they were the
only thing alive, listening for her.

She looked at him finally, gave him a smile that didn't show her
teeth. Her fingers unraveled from his. "You need to shift," she said.
He did, and the car gave a grateful lurch ahead. They drove in silence
the rest of the way home, Stella's soft-shell hands holding tight to her
seat belt.

That night, he was surprised when Stella got into bed next to him in
just a T-shirt. He'd picked up *Cancer Husband*, and found it wasn't
that bad, if a little froufrou for his taste. Of course, he'd started with
the chapter on sex. Very vanilla, but still.

Stella reached out and took the book from his hands. She closed it
without letting him mark his place and dropped it on the floor beside
the bed.

"No more reading," she said.

Hearing her say that made him smile. She used to say that all the time, when she wanted his attention for cuddling, for sex. He rolled toward her. Her body took up less space now—still her, only smaller, like she'd been slightly shrunk. Still the same curves, the waist that hollowed out toward her round hips. He felt huge next to her, a dangerous giant who might roll over and crush her.

Still, he couldn't resist her play. He put his hand softly against her arm, slid it up beneath the shirtsleeve. Her skin was cool, but for the first time in a long time, her muscles didn't tighten in pain at his touch.

"No more reading?" he said. "Why, do you have something better for me to do?"

Stella put her nose against his neck, inhaled deeply.

"I might be able to think of something," she said.

He swallowed hard, unable to speak. How does it feel when your wife comes on to you, finally, finally, after cancer? You feel like the earth has been off its axis, but you didn't notice, until just now, when everything rights itself and settles in, the way it's supposed to be.

"I've missed your body," she said. A sigh, but different from the sighs she'd made in the car. "I've missed *my* body."

How to say he'd missed her body too? He didn't know, so he answered with his fingers on the curve of her hip, followed the slimmed half-circle of her ass. No underwear. The crease where the bottom of her ass met her legs was soft and smooth. Just the feel of it made his hand ache to slap it.

He almost did slap her, but took his hand away, fisted it around the blanket. How could he even think of it? He didn't know, couldn't imagine what kind of person he was to want it the way he did.

Stella's lips moved smooth against his neck. She took his hand from the blankets, put it back on the edge of her hip, where her T-shirt met her skin.

"Undress me," she said.

SHANNA GERMAIN

She sat up, and he pulled her shirt off over her head. And there was her star, just above her right nipple, the red heat of it dulled. He wanted to put his finger on it, to lick it and taste it like sun-warmed earth. He thought it would burn his tongue.

He said, "Does it hurt?"

"Stop asking," she said, and her voice was brisk, but also tired.

He nodded. Even to himself, he'd started to sound like a quiz book. How are you? What do you need? How do you feel? It was like he didn't know what to say if he wasn't asking about her. He searched for something about his own day that would be interesting to her. *I thought about fucking you the way we used to. I thought about clamping your nipples until you cried, until you could sleep and smile again.*

Stella put her own finger over the star, pressed harder than he would have thought.

"Sometimes it hurts," she said. "Not now."

She dropped her hands, put them on his hips.

"Anyway, I don't want to think about it," she said. "Can you just fuck me?"

Her voice was beyond type A into bitter, a spit of bad tastes. It hardened his cock and made him nervous to touch her at the same time. She closed her eyes and leaned her head back, exposing the full length of her soft, white neck, the pulse that talked to him there. He leaned into the pulse, put his lips against the thin blue line.

"Yes," he said. "I can fuck you."

But, then, he couldn't. He wanted to, he tried, but the star kept shining up at him off her skin, a beacon to remind him. Everything he did—his tongue at her pink nipples, avoiding the scar, his fingers down her pale belly, even the moment when, finally, he entered her, every ounce of him inside his cock inside her—at every moment, he was making love, he was taking care. He didn't realize it at the time, he thought they were together in this slow, languid night. But just

157

before he came, he opened his eyes and saw her looking somewhere else. Her body moved in the slow-motion rhythm he'd started, but her mouth made small noises of pain. He tried to rise up off her, but he was already coming, too late to stop and his shudders made his "I'm sorrys" sound tinny and hollow, like they were coming from light-years away.

Stella didn't come on to him again. He wasn't surprised, but he still hoped for it, watched for her to take the lead when she felt okay, but there was nothing. She didn't even undress in front of him.

Within the week, Stella started work again, and they settled back into what he thought of, sadly, as their old rhythm: too much work-work and housework, passing each other on the stairs or in the kitchen, hands full of laundry or dinner. He'd thought that once someone got sick, the way Stella had been sick, you didn't, couldn't, just go back to normal. That you never took each other for granted or passed in the hallway without touching.

He started masturbating in the shower. One hand on his cock, the other against the shower door, just in case she came in to pee. He was embarrassed for himself, for his desire, but he didn't want to embarrass her, or make her feel worse. He used Stella's soap—it smelled of sage, which smelled of her—lathering it until he could slide his fist up and down. Although he tried to think of other things, his mind was all Stella, Stella in nipple clamps, her ass beneath the flat of his hand. Keeping quiet, coming with Stella in the house but without her, made his teeth ache and the bottom of his stomach clench up in cramps. And, still, he couldn't stop. The pain cleansed him somehow, made it safe for him to be around her.

But after two weeks, he couldn't stand not touching her anymore. He put his arms around her one morning while she was dressing and kissed the bare back of her neck. The smell of her sage soap and her curves against the fabric of her skirt made him press his hips into her ass, harder than he'd meant to.

Stella leaned against him, bare shoulder blades pressing into his chest. She let her head fall back onto his shoulder, and he kissed the side of her mouth. He didn't know how much he'd missed her breath, minty and sweet.

"You'll make me late for work," she said against his lips.

"Do you care?" he asked.

She shook her head no, and he turned her toward him, pressed his mouth hard to hers. His hands followed her lower back down to her ass. He cupped his palms around her curves and pulled her hard against him.

Stella made a small cry into his mouth. Panic spread up through his chest. He let go of her body, stepped back and sat on the bed.

"Jesus, Stella, I'm sorry," he said. But even in his panic over hurting her, he couldn't stop looking at her body. How her nipples were like stars too, a constellation against the sky of her chest. How her waist curved in and then swelled into hips. His cock twitched, sending a mixed flood of arousal and shame. Worst husband of the year award, right here.

"Don't you dare," she said. Her voice was shaky. "Don't you fucking dare tell me one more time how sorry you are," she said.

He nodded. His body was heavy, heavy. His hands, his head, his cock shrinking against his thigh, everything held on the bed by this strange gravity. He vowed he would masturbate every day, he would take a lover if he had to. He would not ask anything more of Stella, of her body, than what she offered him.

Stella stepped closer to where he sat. And there was her star, shining with its red heat. He couldn't look away. Did his eyes feel pain? He though they might.

"Touch it," she said.

But he couldn't until she took his wrist and brought his fingers to her skin. The star wasn't hot at all. It felt like Stella's skin, only more so. Thicker, tougher, with six small rays leading out. And she didn't flinch when he pushed a bit against the small points of it. Instead, he thought she might be leaning into him harder.

He pulled his finger away, looked down at it in his lap. Did the tip of it burn, or was it only his guilt that made the skin seem hot? He couldn't tell.

"I don't know what to do," he said.

Stella put her hands beneath her breasts, lifted them up. Her nipples pink stars in their own right. His cock tried to stir, stayed down beneath the weight of air.

"I need you—" Stella started, and then got down on her knees in front of him. There was no rug, and he worried about her knees on the hardwood, but she didn't seem to notice.

"I can only say this once," she said. "Maybe, maybe I can't say it at all."

When Stella tried not to cry, her nose pinkened at the edges. It didn't happen often. He'd seen it once, maybe twice since he'd known her. The splotches of pink made him happy, not because he wanted her to cry, but because he suddenly felt less alone in this thing that had happened.

Stella covered his hands with her own, then lifted her chin until her brown eyes looked right into his.

"I need you to stop fucking me like I'm dying," she said, and her lips moved fast, like she was afraid they would stop. "I'm not dying. But every time you touch me soft, every time you ask if I'm okay, another little piece of me falls off."

Something started within him, a pain he had not known. It began at the inside of his chest, flowed outward to his skin, his arms. His breath hitched and ragged. He wondered if he was having a heart attack. He squeezed Stella's hands, and she squeezed back.

"Now," she said, "I'm going to walk out of the room, and when I come back, I need you to fuck me like I'm actually alive."

Then she stood and turned. Still stuck to the bed, unable to rise or move, he watched her walk out of the room, the strength of her bare back, the way her ass filled out her skirt. The star he couldn't see, but could still feel, not as heat, but as light, guiding him.

"Baby," she said and her voice was strong and sure from out in the hallway, "you're going to have to get out the crocs today."

At the sound of her voice, his body came free of the gravity that held it. He could raise his hands, stand, his cock too rose as high as it could beneath his jeans. Before she came back in, he pulled open the nightstand, dug the nipple clamps from beneath the stack of books they didn't need to read. He looked at the clamps in his hands, their pointy teeth, remembered the contrast their silver shine made against Stella's skin. The way she sighed in release when he clamped them to her nipples. He smiled and slid the clamps beneath the pillow for later. Let her think he'd forgotten, let her wonder. He was the one in charge, after all.

She walked in, naked now, her star shining from its place on her chest. He moved toward her, following its light.

AFTERWORD: THE NEXT STEP

Being kinky is a life-long journey, one that has the potential to take you to amazing places and to bring you to incredible heights. New pleasures and experiences are always just around the next bend—and now you have a wide array of tools and tips to go on the kinky adventure of a lifetime.

No matter what elements of kink get you off or turn you on, it's time to get out there and enjoy both the journey and the destination. Time to take the next step toward your kinky self and become as kinky as you wanna be.

LEARNING THE LANGUAGE:
A GLOSSARY OF KINK

This isn't a comprehensive list of the language of BDSM—consider it more of a starter set of important words, phrases and concepts. Because language is a living thing, the meaning of it is ever changing, and it may vary from place to place and kink culture to kink culture.

Choose the words that best suit your self-definition and your worldview, but be open to the idea that others will not use the same words to mean the same thing. As always, clear communication is the key to safe, arousing kink.

BDSM Basics

Every culture has its code words—its shibboleths if you will—and the BDSM culture is no exception. Here are some basic, commonly used terms to get you speaking the language of lust.

Aftercare: A space of time post-BDSM scene or play session during which the participants "return to reality." Often, this time is used for discussing the experience of the scene, exploring physical or emotional reactions and dealing with any possible concerns.

BDSM: Bondage/Discipline, Dominance/Submission, Sadism/Masochism: while this combined acronym means different things to different people, it's most commonly used to refer to anything and everything within the kink community.

Bottom: In its most basic form, the term typically means the person who is receiving the action (in contrast to the top, who is the person doing the action). Can also be used to mean the person who has given up control or power.

Collared: A submissive, slave, or puppy who is owned.

Collaring: The formal ceremony or agreement in which a dominant commits to a submissive.

Consent: A mutual agreement (between two or more people) to the terms of a BDSM scene or relationship.

Consensual Nonconsensuality: A mutual agreement (between two or more people) that within defined limits, consent is given without knowledge of the actions planned. Typically used only between partners who know each other well or who have otherwise set out clear safe limits ahead of time.

Contract: A written agreement between two or more people (typically between a dominant and submissive). It typically outlines the agreed-upon structure, rules and boundaries of the relationship.

Dominant/Dom/Domme/Dominatrix: Any number of terms for a person who exercises control. The former two may be used with either gender, while the latter two are most often used with women.

Fetish: A specific obsession, delight, or interest in one type of experience, object or activity.

Good pain and bad pain: Pleasant pain versus unpleasant pain. The first typically refers to consensual pain that is a positive, desired part of a BDSM experience, while the second is not.

Limits: Lines that someone is hesitant to cross or will not cross. The term "hard limits" defines the non-negotiable "nos"—what someone will absolutely not do—while "soft limits" refer to something that someone is hesitant about.

Masochist: Someone who enjoys receiving pain for sensual or sexual pleasure.

Master/slave: A consensual relationship in which one person (the slave) gives control to another (the Master).

Pain slut: A person who enjoys receiving a heavy degree of pain but may or may not necessarily enjoy submitting.

Risk aware consensual kink (RACK): A tenet used by some BDSM practitioners to determine the appropriateness and safety of BDSM play. The philosophy encourages all participants to understand that there are inherent risks to kink, to be well informed of what those risks are and to give and get informed consent before engaging in any BDSM activity.

Sadism: Sexual enjoyment from hurting or punishing someone.

Sadist: A person who enjoys inflicting pain, usually sexually.

Safe, sane and consensual (SSC): A tenet used by some BDSM practitioners to determine the appropriateness and safety of BDSM play.

Safeword: A code word that can be used to stop any form of BDSM activity.

Sensation play: BDSM play where the intent is to push people's sensory limits, thus exploring texture, sensory deprivation, and on through to whips, flagellation and edgeplay.

Slave: A person (usually submissive) who consensually gives up control of some aspect(s) of his or her life to another person (usually the master).

Switch: A person who alternates their role from experience to experience or even within the same play sessions. A switch may consider herself to be both dominant and submissive or neither, depending on her mood and play partners.

Top: In its most basic form, the term typically means the person who is doing the action (in contrast to the bottom, who is the person receiving the action). Can also be used to mean the person who has the control or power.

Vanilla: A person or act that is not typically thought of as kinky, or does not include BDSM activity.

Fetishes and Interests

Again, this isn't an all-encompassing list of things that kinky people like to do in their bedrooms, on their lawns or in the neighborhood dungeon. That alone would take a whole book. Instead, I've pulled out some of the more common fetishes, along with a few other terms that are either often misunderstood or aren't self-explanatory.

Abrasion: Stimulating the skin with abrasive materials such as sandpaper, rough leather, sex toys, et cetera.

Age play: Acting as if you were either younger or older than you really are. Examples include Daddy/daughter, mommy/baby, and teacher/student role-play.

Anal play: Play where the anus is stimulated and/or penetrated with fingers, fist, beads, dildos, anal plus or penis.

Anal torture: Inflicting pain on the anus.

Animal play: Acting or dressing like an animal, such as a dog, cat or pony.

Ball stretching: Play that involves attaching weights to the testicles and scrotum in order to provide sensations such as discomfort and pain.

Bathroom use control: Play where the dominant controls the submissive's bodily functions in some ways. This can include enemas, diapers, and catheterization.

Beating: Striking various parts of the body with an object or hand. Depending on the instrument used, can also be called spanking, whipping or caning.

Being serviced: Play in which the dominant provides instructions to the submissive on how to perform sexually.

Biting: Play that involves biting, typically to induce pain. Bite play that causes broken skin or bleeding can be dangerous and should be done with caution.

Bondage: Play involving the physical restraint of a partner in some fashion. This can range from handcuffs to breast bondage to total body restraint.

Breast bondage: A type of bondage that focuses specifically on the breasts.

Breath control: Play in which breathing is controlled in some fashion. This is a controversial topic within the BDSM community due to the potential for injury and death.

Caning: An advanced type of painful beating administered to the fleshy part of the buttocks with a cane.

Catheterization: Play where a flexible medical tube is inserted into the area controlled by the bladder. Typically used for bathroom use control.

Chastity: Play that involves denying individuals sexual access to their genitals without explicit permission from their partner. This may be done with a device, such as a chastity belt or cock cage, or through power exchanges.

Cock and ball torture (CBT): Play that involves the torture of the male genitals for sexual gratification.

Edgeplay: A wide, subjective definition for play that involves a chance of physical or emotional harm. Edgeplay means different things to different people, but commonly accepted forms of edgeplay include knife play, gunplay, breath play, and blood play.

Enemas: A type of bathroom use control or medical play that involves a thorough anal cleaning.

Erotic sexual denial: Play that keeps someone in a continual state of arousal with delayed release.

Erotic spanking: Spanking another person for the sexual arousal or gratification of either or both parties.

Exhibitionism: A type of fetish or activity marked by the act of exposing oneself in public or private.

Face slapping: Play that involves a moderate amount of slapping or hitting of the face, typically to exert humiliation or control.

Fellatio: Oral sex performed on a penis.

Fisting: Play that involves attempting to place the entire hand into the rectum or vagina. This type of play requires extreme care, trust and patience, and should be properly studied before attempting.

Food play or forced feeding: Play where a dominant controls the amount and type of food and drink that a submission is allowed to consume.

Foot worship: Play that involves a fetish for feet. Boot worship, high heel domination and stocking fetishes are also sometimes included in this phrase.

Forced [fill in the blank]: Almost any type of play can have the word *forced* added to the beginning of it and it will become a BDSM act: forced feeding, forced homosexuality, forced masturbation, forced smoking. Typically enacted between a dominant and a submissive, and accompanied by a loss of control and sense of humiliation.

Genitorture: Play that involves any type of torture of the genitals.

Golden showers: Play that includes the act of urinating on, or being urinated on by, another person.

Hair pulling: Tugging or yanking someone's hair for the purpose of inducing pain, proving dominance or causing humiliation.

Hand jobs: The act of using your hands on a man's penis to create pleasure, consensual pain and/or orgasm.

Humiliation: Play designed to humiliate submissives by requiring them to do something they normally wouldn't do. Public sex, wearing certain types of clothing, or playing out scenes can all be forms of humiliation play.

Ice play: Using ice or other frozen objects on the nipples, genitals or skin.

Impact play: A type of sensation play that focuses on the impact of whips, crops, paddles and floggers against the skin.

Knife play: Considered to be a type of abrasion play, blood play and edgeplay, knife play involves cutting the skin with sharp objects for pain, sensation and decorative scarring.

Medical scenes: Role-play that replicates a doctor's office. It can include exams, needle play and more.

Needle play: Piercings done with sterile needles, typically temporary.

Over the knee spanking (OTK): Just what it sounds like. Can include role-play such as teacher/student and Daddy/daughter, and provides sensation, pain and humiliation.

Pussy worship: The practice of erotic play that involves worshipping someone's pussy through licking, cleaning, shaving and other activities.

Ponygirl or ponyboy: A submissive who acts and dresses in a pony outfit, including a bit and an anal plug with a tail.

Puppy: A submissive who acts like a puppy by barking, eating from a bowl, sleeping on the floor, et cetera.

Rape fantasy: This broad term encompasses many aspects of rape fantasies, including daydreaming about being involved in consensual rape-play.

Fantasy rape: Type of play where rape fantasies are fulfilled in a safe, consensual environment. Aftercare is extremely important in this type of play.

Rimming: Kissing, licking or otherwise using your mouth around the rectal area.

Spanking: This all-encompassing term includes striking someone with the flat of the hand, a paddle, a hairbrush, a riding crop, et cetera, on the butt to induce pain, pleasure, submission, punishment or humiliation.

Scat play: Feces play.

Voyeurism: The act of watching someone else engage in kinky activities for your own pleasure (and possibly for theirs, if they are exhibitionists).

Toys and Objects

There are far more toys available to you than I've listed here, but these are some great ones to get you started. Some of them you've probably heard of many times, but others might be new to you.

Anal beads: A set of strung beads used to insert into the anus to stimulate the anal nerves as foreplay or to cause orgasm.

Blindfold: Anything that can be used to block someone's sense of sight and provide heightened sensory experiences.

Butt plug: A toy with a flared base that is designed to be inserted into the anus. They are made for both men and women, can be made from a variety of materials and may vibrate.

Cock ring: A rubber, metal or leather ring that is strapped around the base of the penis, or around the penis and scrotum.

Collar: Typically made of leather, rubber or metal, and worn around the neck to indicate that someone is a submissive or that he is "owned" by someone.

Cuffs: A bondage device used to hold the wrists or ankles, typically made of leather or metal.

Dildo: A phallic-shaped toy that is designed to be inserted into the body, typically made from latex, glass or wood.

Flogger: A whip-like device with many tails that is used to cause increased sensation on the butt, back or genitals.

Gag: Anything that can be used to restrict the use of the mouth, including ball gags, cloth and leather.

Nipple clamps: Closing devices that can be placed on the nipples to cause pain, pleasure and additional sensations.

Riding crop: A short whip with a loop on the end that is used in pony play, as well as for spanking, punishment, and humiliation.

Strap-on: A device or harness used to hold a dildo in place.

Vibrator: A vibrating toy that comes in a variety of shapes and sizes, which is used for stimulation, pleasure and orgasm.

Public Play

Whether you're interested in attending a nonsexual gathering of fellow kinksters or want to head off to the local kink club, here are some phrases to get you started.

Dungeon: A public or private room or designated play space filled with BDSM equipment.

Dungeon monitor: Commonly called a DM, this person supervises the participants at play parties, dungeon events or other activities to ensure safety, enforce house rules and answer questions.

Handkerchief codes: Visible signs to indicate to others your area of BDSM interest; a color worn on the left indicates a top, on the right indicates a bottom. Less commonly used than they used to be.

Munch: A group of kinky people meeting in a home, club, restaurant or other nonsexual space.

Play party: An event that involves people and couples engaging in BDSM activities.

Scene: A specific time period during which one or more BDSM activities take place. Typically followed up by aftercare.

Swapping: Switching partners for play purposes, usually for a set period of time or to partake in a specific activity.

RESOURCE GUIDE

Nonfiction

Books

Come Hither: A Commonsense Guide To Kinky Sex, by Gloria G. Brame (New York: Touchstone, 2000).

The Compleat Slave: Creating and Living an Erotic Dominant/Submissive Lifestyle, by Jack Rinella (Los Angeles: Daedalus Publishing, 1992).

Consensual Sadomasochism: How To Talk About It and Do It Safely, by William A. Henkin, PhD and Sybil Holiday, CCSSE (Los Angeles: Daedalus Publishing, 1996).

Conquer Me: girl-to-girl wisdom about fulfilling your submissive desires, by Kacie Cunningham (Eugene, OR: Greenery Press, 2010).

Different Loving: A Complete Exploration of the World of Sexual Dominance and Submission, by Gloria G. Brame, Jon Jacobs, and William D. Brame (New York: Villard Books, 1993).

Domination & Submission: The BDSM Relationship Handbook, by Michael Makai (Amazon Digital Services, 2013).

Dungeon Emergencies and Supplies, by Jay Wiseman (Oakland: Greenery Press, 2004).

Family Jewels: A Guide to Male Genital Play and Torment, by Hardy Haberman (Oakland: Greenery Press, 2001).

Fetish Sex: An Erotic Guide for Couples, by Violet Blue (Los Angeles: Daedalus Publishing, 2006).

The Master's Manual: A Handbook of Erotic Dominance, by Jack Rinella

(Los Angeles: Daedalus Publishing, 1994).

Miss Abernathy's Concise Slave Training Manual, by Christina Abernathy (Oakland: Greenery Press, 1996).

The Mistress Manual: The Good Girl's Guide to Female Dominance, by Mistress Lorelei (Oakland: Greenery Press, 2000).

The New Bottoming Book, by Dossie Easton and Janet Hardy (Oakland: Greenery Press, 2011).

The New Topping Book, by Dossie Easton and Janet Hardy (Oakland: Greenery Press, 2011).

Partners in Power: Living in Kinky Relationships, by Jack Rinella (Oakland: Greenery Press, 2003).

Playing Well with Others: Your Field Guide to Discovering, Exploring and Navigating the Kink, Leather and BDSM Communities, by Lee Harrington and Mollena Williams (Oakland: Greenery Press, 2012).

Screw the Roses, Send Me the Thorns: The Romance and Sexual Sorcery of Sadomasochism, by Philip Miller and Molly Devon (Fairfield, CT: Mystic Rose Books, 1995).

The Seductive Art of Japanese Bondage, by Midori (Oakland: Greenery Press, 2002).

Sensuous Magic: A Guide for Adventurous Couples, by Patrick Califia (Berkeley: Cleis Press, 1993).

SM 101: A Realistic Introduction, by Jay Wiseman (Eugene, OR: Greenery Press, 1998).

Two Knotty Boys Showing You the Ropes: A Step-by-Step, Illustrated Guide for Tying Sensual and Decorative Rope Bondage, by Two Knotty Boys (San Francisco: Green Candy Press, 2007).

The Ultimate Guide to Kink: BDSM, Role Play and the Erotic Edge, by Tristan Taormino (Berkeley: Cleis Press, 2012).

When Someone You Love Is Kinky, by Dossie Easton and Catherine Liszt (Eugene, OR: Greenery Press, 2000).

Videos

The Expert Guide to Sensual Bondage with Midori, directed by Tristan Taormino (Vivid-Ed).

Nina Hartley's Guide Series. Nina Hartley hosts and Ernest Greene directs this DVD series covering domination, submission, bondage sex, spanking, and more (Adam and Eve).

Penny Flame's Expert Guide to Rough Sex, directed by Tristan Taormino (Vivid-Ed).

The S/M Arts Collection: The Pain Game & Tie Me Up, hosted by Cleo Dubois (Academy of S/M Arts).

Fiction

Books

Anything for You: Erotica for Kinky Couples, edited by Rachel Kramer Bussel (Berkeley: Cleis Press, 2012).

Best Bondage Erotica series (Berkeley: Cleis Press).

Bondage on a Budget, edited by Alison Tyler (Point Reyes, CA: Pretty Things Press, 2002).

Bound by Lust: Romantic Stories of Submission and Sensuality, edited by Shanna Germain (Berkeley: Cleis Press, 2012).

The Big Book of Bondage: Sexy Tales of Erotic Restraint, edited by Alison Tyler (Berkeley: Cleis Press, 2012).

The Marketplace (3rd ed.), by Laura Antoniou (Cambridge: Circlet Press, 2010).

Serving Him: Sexy Stories of Submission, edited by Rachel Kramer Bussel (Berkeley: Cleis Press, 2013).

Slave to Love: Erotic Stories of Bondage and Desire, edited by Alison Tyler (Berkeley: Cleis Press, 2011).

Spanked: Red Cheeked Erotica, edited by Rachel Kramer Bussel (Berkeley: Cleis Press, 2008).

Surrender: Erotic Tales of Female Pleasure and Submission, edited by
  Rachel Kramer Bussel (Berkeley: Cleis Press, 2011).
Sweet Danger: Erotic Stories of Forbidden Desire for Couples, edited by
  Violet Blue (Berkeley: Cleis Press, 2011).

Movies
9 1/2 Weeks
Belle de Jour
Flower and Snake
Preaching to the Perverted
Quills
Secretary
The Story of O
Tie Me Up! Tie Me Down!
Walk All Over Me

ABOUT THE CONTRIBUTORS

JANINE ASHBLESS (janineashbless.blogspot.com) has had nine books of erotica published by Black Lace, Samhain and others. Her short stories have appeared in many Cleis Press anthologies, including three volumes of the Best Women's Erotica series. She's currently writing Cleis an erotic romance trilogy about fallen angels: the first, *Cover Him with Darkness*, published 2014.

RACHEL KRAMER BUSSEL (rachelkramerbussel.com) is the editor of *Anything for You: Erotica for Kinky Couples; Cheeky Spanking Stories; Bottoms Up; Spanked; Please, Sir; Please, Ma'am; Baby Got Back: Anal Erotica; The Big Book of Orgasms; Lust in Latex; Suite Encounters; Irresistible* and many other books.

LEE HARRINGTON (PassionAndSoul.com) is an internationally known spiritual and erotic authenticity educator, gender explorer, eclectic artist and author/editor on human erotic and sacred experience. His books include *Shibari You Can Use: Japanese Rope Bondage and Erotic Macramé, Sacred Kink: The Eightfold Paths of BDSM and Beyond*, and many more.

As happily self-identified pervert, **STELLA HARRIS** (stellaharris. net) has a passion for BDSM education. Through her writing and teaching she explores the complex world of love and lust and strives to help people explore their kinks safely and free of shame.

SHANNA KATZ, M.Ed, ACS (ShannaKatz.com), author of *Your Pleasure Map, Oral Sex That'll Blow Her Mind* and *Lesbian Sex Positions,* is a queer kinky disabled feisty femme board-certified sexologist, sexuality educator and professional pervert who's using her master's of sexuality education to provide accessible, open-source sex education to people around the country.

DR. LYNK is a doctor of physical therapy and certified strength and conditioning specialist.

KRISTINA LLOYD's (kristinalloyd.co.uk) five novels, including *Undone,* are published by Black Lace and her short stories have appeared in dozens of anthologies. She has a master's degree in twentieth-century literature and lives in Brighton, U.K.

NIKKI MAGENNIS (nikkimagennis.com) is an author, poet and artist. She lives in Scotland between the forests and the sea and can never quite let herself be tied down to one or the other.

SUNNY MEGATRON (sunnymegatron.com) is a sex and BDSM educator, blogger, and pleasure advocate. She teaches sexuality, relationship, and kink workshops across the U.S. with her partner, Ken Melvoin-Berg. Her current project is hosting the sexual health and wellness web series Outside the Box.

REMITTANCE GIRL (remittancegirl.com) is the pen name of Madeleine Morris. Author of numerous published short stories, three novellas and one novel, Madeleine has been writing erotica for more than a decade. She holds an MA in writing and is working toward a PhD in creative writing.

TERESA NOELLE ROBERTS writes sexy stories for lusty romantics of all persuasions. Her work appears in *Best Bondage Erotica 2014, The Big Book of Bondage, Mammoth Book of Best New Erotica 12, Best Erotic Romance 2013* and other provocatively titled anthologies. Look for her BDSM and erotic paranormal romance novels.

DONNA GEORGE STOREY (DonnaGeorgeStorey.com) is the author of *Amorous Woman,* an erotic novel based on her experiences living in Japan, and a column for the *Erotica Readers and Writers* blog. Her stories have appeared in *Penthouse, The Mammoth Book of Erotica Presents the Best of Donna George Storey* and *Bound by Lust.*

CECILIA TAN (blog.ceciliatan.com) writes about her passions from her home in the Boston area. The founder of Circlet Press, she is also the author of many books (*Slow Surrender, The Prince's Boy, Mind Games,* et cetera) and the recipient of many awards both for her writing and her BDSM activism.

JAY WISEMAN (jaywiseman.com) is the author of the best-selling and internationally distributed book *SM 101: A Realistic Introduction.* He is also the author of *Jay Wiseman's Erotic Bondage Handbook* and *Dungeon Emergencies and Supplies.* He is active as an author, video producer, presenter, workshop leader, activist and expert witness.

KRISTINA WRIGHT is the editor of over a dozen anthologies for Cleis Press, including the Best Erotic Romance series. She holds degrees in English and humanities and her short fiction has appeared in dozens of anthologies. She lives in Virginia with her husband and their two young sons.

ABOUT THE AUTHOR

SHANNA GERMAIN (vorpalblonde.com) claims the titles of wanderluster, flower picker, tire kicker, knife licker, she-devil, vorpal blonde and Schrödinger's brat.

With a whole lot of writing years under her belt (or her collar, depending on the day), Shanna's poems, essays, short stories, novellas, articles and more have found homes in hundreds of magazines, newspapers, books and websites.

An associate fellow at the Attic Institute in Portland, OR, she has taught classes in writing, publishing, media and photography at a wide variety of places. She's even garnered an award here and there, including a Pushcart nomination, the Rauxa Prize for Erotic Poetry and the C. Hamilton Bailey Poetry Fellowship. She keeps her ego in a tiny glass jar and feeds it drops of seawater and baby crickets so that it will never outgrow its cage.